FASCIAL
FITNESS

ROBERT SCHLEIP

with Johanna Bayer

The English language first edition first published in 2017. This second edition published in 2021 by
Lotus Publishing
Apple Tree Cottage, Inlands Road, Nutbourne, Chichester, PO18 8RJ
North Atlantic Books
Huichin, unceded Ohlone land
Berkeley, California

Fascial Fitness: Practical Exercises to Stay Flexible, Active and Pain Free in Just 20 Minutes a Week, Second Edition, is sponsored and published by North Atlantic Books, an educational non-profit based on the unceded Ohlone land Huichin (Berkeley, CA), that collaborates with partners to develop cross-cultural perspectives, nurture holistic views of art, science, the humanities, and healing, and seed personal and global transformation by publishing work on the relationship of body, spirit, and nature.

North Atlantic Books' publications are distributed to the US trade and internationally by Penguin Random House Publishers Services. For further information, visit our website at www.northatlanticbooks.com.

Important note
The content of this book has been researched and carefully verified to the best knowledge and belief of the authors and publisher, against sources they consider to be trustworthy. Nevertheless, this book is not intended as a substitute for individual fitness, nutritional and medical advice. If you wish to seek medical advice, please consult a qualified physician. The publisher and the authors shall not be liable for any negative effects directly or indirectly associated with the information given in this book.

Editor: Simone Fischer
Cover design: Pamela Machleidt
Cover images: Vukašin Latinović, Graphics: shutterstock/fox_industry
Models: Martina Meinl, Markus Rossmann
Layout: Medlar Publishing Solutions Pvt Ltd, India
Typesetting: Satzwerk Huber, Germering, Melanie Kitt, Lisa Killer
Printing: Kultur Sanat Printing House, Turkey

British Library of Cataloguing-in-Publication Data
A CIP record for this book is available from the British Library
ISBN 978 1 913088 21 7 (Lotus Publishing)
ISBN 978 1 62317 674 7 (North Atlantic Books)

Library of Congress Cataloguing-in-Publication Data
Names: Schleip, Robert, author. | Bayer, Johanna, other.
Title: Fascial fitness : practical exercises to stay flexible, active and
    pain free in just 20 minutes a week / Robert Schleip with Johanna Bayer.
Description: Second edition. | Berkeley : North Atlantic Books / Lotus
    Publishing, [2021] | "The best-selling guide, expanded and revised" --
    title page. | Includes bibliographical references and index.
Identifiers: LCCN 2020054558 (print) | LCCN 2020054559 (ebook) | ISBN
    9781623176747 (trade paperback) | ISBN 9781623176754 (ebook)
Subjects: LCSH: Fasciae (Anatomy) | Connective tissues. | Exercise. |
    Movement therapy.
Classification: LCC QM563 .S35 2021 (print) | LCC QM563 (ebook) | DDC
    611/.74--dc23
LC record available at https://lccn.loc.gov/2020054558
LC ebook record available at https://lccn.loc.gov/2020054559

ROBERT SCHLEIP

with Johanna Bayer

FASCIAL FITNESS

Practical Exercises to Stay Flexible, Active and Pain Free in Just 20 Minutes a Week

Second Edition

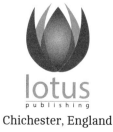

lotus
publishing
Chichester, England

North Atlantic Books
Huichin, unceded Ohlone land
Berkeley, California

Contents

Foreword 6
by Klaus Eder

Foreword to the revised
2018 edition 10
by Robert Schleip

Introduction:
Why you need to exercise
your fascia 15
A journey into the undiscovered
    world of fascia 20

Chapter 1:
Fascia and connective
tissue – what are they? 23

Fresh fascia 24
The basic building block with many
    functions 25
The components of fascia 26
Types and functions of connective
    tissue 30
A new way of looking at the body . . 32
The four basic functions of fascia . . 33
Severing ties with invasive surgery 35
High performance: fascia and
    the musculoskeletal system 36
Information centres: fascia as
    a sensory organ 39
An unusual case: Ian Waterman –
    the man who couldn't feel his body 42
The science of fascia 43
Fascial pioneers: Alfred Pischinger
    and his system of basic regulation 44
Fascial pioneers: Elisabeth Dicke
    and connective tissue massage 46
Fascial pioneers: Ida Rolf, founder
    of Rolfing therapy and structural
    integration 49
Fascial pioneers: Andrew Taylor Still,
    the founder of osteopathy 51

New perspectives on back
    pain – the suffering we share 53

Chapter 2:
The principles of
fascia training 57

Healthy movement in
    everyday life 58
What you need to know before
    you train 60
How the muscles and fascia
    work together 61
Fascial lines and the tension
    network 67
How does connective tissue
    respond to training? 78
Everything you need to know
    about fascia training 85
Not an automatic process:
    muscle and fascia training 87
Stretching and training: what
    fascia needs 88
The four dimensions of
    fascia training 102
Before we begin: which tissue
    type are you? 113
Tests to determine types of
    connective tissue 120

Chapter 3:
The exercises 131

What do you need? 133
Clothing and shoes 136
Things to consider before
    you begin 136
Your guide: the four dimensions
    of fascia training 138
Mindful breathing to support your
    training 140

The basic program 142

Exercises for problem areas:
back, neck, arms, hips and feet . . 156
A short program for back
    problems 157
Office pains: problems in the
    neck, arms and shoulders 168
The hip area 176
For the feet and gait 183

For Vikings, contortionists
and crossover types 191
Vikings with firm connective
    tissue 192
Contortionists with soft connective
    tissue 195
Crossover types 197

Different exercises for men
and women 199
Exercises and tips for women 200
Exercises and tips for men 204

Exercises for athletes 210
Sport-specific fascial care 211
Self-help for muscle soreness 212
Balancing exercises for runners . . . 217
Tips for cyclists 220

Everyday life as an exercise:
making your movements
more creative 221

Guidelines for the elderly 225

Chapter 4:
Fascia, physiotherapy and
gentle methods of recovery 229

Yoga then and now 231
Classic massage and manual
    therapy 236
Acupuncture 237
Rolfing therapy 238
Osteopathy 239
Pilates 241

In check: new fascial trends 242

Chapter 5:
Fascial fitness: healthy
eating and lifestyle 253

Maintaining a healthy weight 254
No smoking! 254
Staying hydrated 255
Getting enough protein 256
Vitamin C for collagen 257
Zinc, copper, magnesium and
    potassium for fitness 257
Getting enough sleep 259
From silica to gelatine – what
    supplements should we
    be taking? 259
The great sugar debate 262
Inflammation and fascia 263
Tips from me to you 265

Chapter 6:
Periodised fascia training
for speed, power and injury
resilience 267
Bill Parisi & Johnathon Allen

Fascia training 101 270
Vector variability 272
Odd position strength 274
Power and speed 275
Speed, agility and quickness 277
Rest and recovery 278
References 280

The future is fascial! 283

Appendix
About the authors 286
Further reading, additional links
    and recommended suppliers 288
Photo credits 289
Overview of exercises 290
Index 292

Foreword

by Klaus Eder

When I was invited to write a foreword to this book in 2014, I couldn't possibly turn it down. Fascia is my favourite subject, and one that I have been dealing with throughout my entire career – initially without knowing a great deal about it; only having a sense of its importance and noticing it during treatment. Thankfully that's all now changed, both for myself and almost everyone else in the same position – especially since the publication of *Fascial Fitness* Dr Robert Schleip, which he wrote together with science author Johanna Bayer. This clear, concise book has become an essential resource and one that can be found on my own bookshelf and those of many of my colleagues. It is also something I often recommend to my patients and clients.

I hold the work of Robert Schleip in the highest possible regard, not least due to his commitment to sharing his practical knowledge and understanding of fascia. The two of us have long been united by a fascination with the role of fascia in the human body and how this affects us, especially in the field of sports medicine. Thanks to his research, along with his engagement in the field of physiotherapy,

over the last 15 years Robert Schleip has succeeded not only in bringing fascia to the scientific community, but also in making it the focal point of sports physiotherapy and manual therapy. He also made the subject accessible to the general public and has proven himself to be a remarkable talent with his fascinating talks, seminars, workshops, training programs for amateur athletes and, of course, his best-selling books.

Words cannot express how happy I am that this clear, accessible book on fascia and fascial exercises has achieved so much success – but with almost 80,000 copies sold, the numbers speak for themselves. Robert Schleip has succeeded in bringing the latest findings on fascia to the broadest of readerships, making it accessible to many different people.

The publication of these findings has also been just as beneficial – if not more so – to the professional field in which I have spent most of my career. I have been working with top athletes for the past few decades. These sportspeople trust me to look after their bodies. I have been taking care of the German national football team since 1988 and have supported 'our boys' through eight World Cups, eight European Championships and ten Olympic Games. From 1990 until 2012, I was also in the fortunate position of working

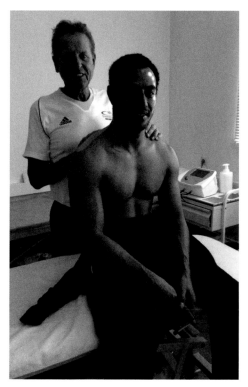

At the Winter Olympics in Sochi in 2014, I also treated Bruno Banani, a luge athlete from Tonga.

for the German Davis Cup tennis team as their physiotherapist. My approach to diagnosing and treating athletes is achieved using only my bare hands. This way, I get to know the consistency of most of the athletes' muscles and fascia like the back of my own hand. I know only too well the major personal challenges players face when they have to retire temporarily or permanently as a result of injury or overused muscles – and I can say with confidence that the fascia is almost always affected. In the majority of cases, I am able to reduce the severity of the pain and shorten their period of downtime. What helps me the most under these circumstances is my knowledge of fascial anatomy and my many years of experience as a physiotherapist.

However, the way I and other therapists practiced in this field was for a long time based more on intuition and experience than on any concrete knowledge. The fundamental change came as a result of the scientific work of Dr Robert Schleip. With their experiments, he and his colleagues at the University of Ulm have added a whole new basis to the understanding of fascia. They showed that fascia can harden the muscles independently and that this can also happen as a result of stress.

As a manual therapist, for many decades I have been able to feel these lumps with my fingers when treating athletes and other patients. Yet I often fell short when it came to describing or explaining them – I didn't have any concrete knowledge, only my intuition. When talking to orthopaedic surgeons and medical professionals, however, I quickly realised that they had very definite opinions about the origin of these lumps, and these opinions did not fit in with my intuition as a practitioner. Those discussions proved to be far from easy.

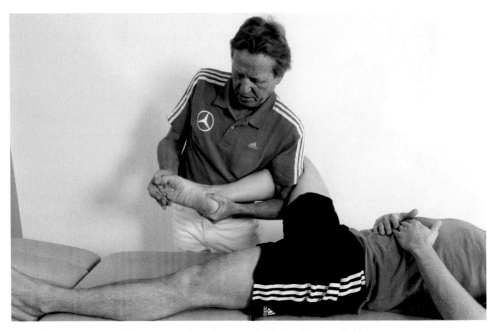

At my clinic in Donaustauf, Germany, I primarily use methods that focus on fascia.

This is no longer the case, with fascia now incorporated into diagnosis and treatment as a matter of course. It was Robert Schleip who made that happen, and on an international scale. He cannot be commended highly enough for this work. In 2006, he received the prestigious Vladimir Janda Award for Musculoskeletal Medicine for his innovative biological studies. I had the pleasure of getting to know Professor Janda, the great muscle researcher and neurophysiologist from Prague, personally. He was one of the first to point out to myself and other pioneers in the field of modern sports physiotherapy how important fascia is for the process of healthy movement and how remarkably it responds to treatment. This is something I have observed not only with my top athletes, but also with the amateur sports enthusiasts that we have been treating for many years at our Eden Reha treatment centre in Donaustauf.

I therefore very much welcome the fact that this book is currently being revised and reissued to incorporate the latest knowledge and understanding that has been gained since 2014. So much has happened in the intervening years – not least thanks to the international work of Robert Schleip – that there is a great deal of excitement within the therapist community about what the two authors are currently putting together.

In my view, the specialised fascia training that Robert Schleip and his colleagues have developed in recent years – and continuously refine – has huge potential. It would make me very happy if this new edition means that even more people can have fun and get results when exercising, without becoming injured or having to rely on therapeutic help from me and my fellow fascia specialists. As sports therapists, we need not fear that we will be out of a job, but rather – thanks to the global network of researchers that Robert Schleip has created in recent years – our work will be easier for us in the future.

Klaus Eder
Donaustauf, June 2018

Klaus Eder is a physiotherapist and has worked for many years with top athletes and Olympians who practice many different kinds of sport, such as the German national football team and the German Davis Cup team. He runs Eden Reha in Donaustauf – a practice for physiotherapy and remedial gymnastics along with an affiliated rehabilitation clinic for sports and accident injuries. Eden Reha also offers ongoing training for physicians, health professionals and sports coaches, covering topics such as sports physiotherapy and fascia therapy.

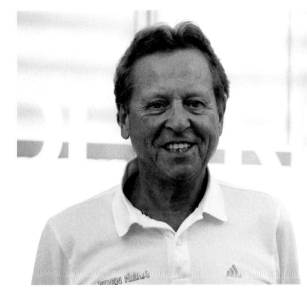

Foreword to the revised 2018 edition

by Robert Schleip

The great wave of interest in fascia began in Germany at the end of 2012. Following news reports on major national television channels, myself and my Fascia Research Team at Ulm University were inundated with inquiries. Some of these queries came from journalists, but we were mostly being approached by athletes, trainers, instructors, physiotherapists, researchers,

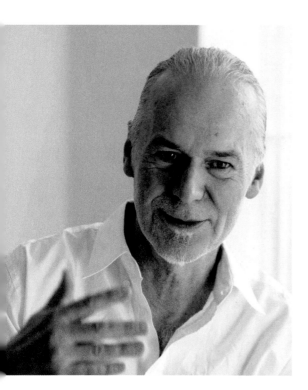

doctors, clinics and associations. To this day, this fascination with fascia has not abated. Practically every adult education centre across the whole of Germany offers a course on fascia training as part of its program, and there is hardly a health or sports editor in the country who hasn't covered the topic at some point. Almost all training systems, from fitness to yoga, also involve fascia.

That is largely down to this little book, which was first published in autumn 2014. There are now eight editions and over 100,000 copies have been sold – a level of success that I could never have anticipated. We have also seen a surprising level of international demand. Since 2014, *Fascial Fitness* has been published in English, Taiwanese, Chinese and Korean, with other languages set to follow. The huge number of guides and books on fascia, many of which took our book as a model, show just how much interest there is in the topic.

Equally, the scientific research into fascia has also come on in leaps and bounds since 2014. There are now so many reputable publications in high-quality journals worldwide that even die-hard critics from the fields of medical and sports science field have had to acknowledge how much they underestimated the importance of fascia and the potential of targeted fascia training.

Many more institutes and researchers are now focusing on fascia, which is an even greater incentive for anyone working in this area to keep fascia in their sights. After all, this connective tissue still has many secrets that are yet to be revealed. Equally, it is precisely this scientific side of the latest research into fascia that enables us to put the new findings into practice: in sport, physiotherapy, medicine and rehabilitation, as well as in our home and work lives – in relation to occupational health, for example.

Of course, not everything we know about fascia is new. What is new, however, is the scientific phase that we are in now. Many of the methods we are now using are also new, such as those borrowed from molecular biology. We also have new devices and imaging processes at our disposal, such as ultrasound elastography, which we are currently using as part of a pilot project in Ulm. The greatest turn up for the books, however, is the new approach to fascial research – that of interdisciplinary perspectives and international collaboration. Fascia conferences bring together academic researchers, physicians and scientists to exchange ideas with physiotherapists, massage therapists and trainers. Our fourth International Fascia Research Congress held in Washington, D.C. in 2015 paid testament to the great global interest and aspirational mindset that now exists across many disciplines. Our next Fascia

Research Congress took place with over 1000 international participants in Berlin in September 2018. And here at the University of Ulm, we have since held our second conference on the topic of 'Connective tissue in sports medicine', where we brought together leading international researchers in the field.

What I enjoy most about these developments is that they provide a platform for fascia researchers – all working in different disciplines and countries around the world – to meet face-to-face for lively discussions on their specialist subject. This is something that simply didn't happen before. Up to now, there has been a strict separation between the different disciplines, while today scientists are able to benefit from practitioners and vice versa. The process we are currently going through in terms of training methods and practice is a completely normal part of developing new systems. The outcomes of new research are used to devise concrete applications, and the principles are converted into methods and tested out – often even before there has been adequate scientific investigation. In doing so, we proceed according to reasonable assumptions and plausibility, and ensure the best progress by relying on the research results already available. Many training methods have been developed in this way. Athletes and coaches would receive ideas and

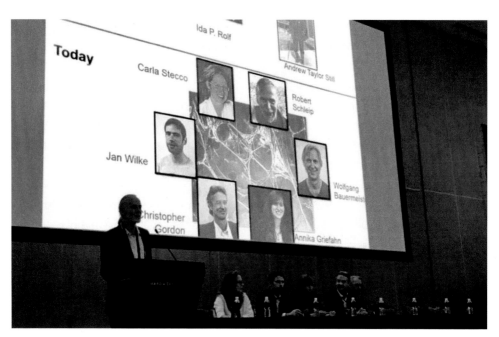

Fascia has become a novel topic of plenary sessions in many international congresses; here at the 9th Interdisciplinary World Congress on Low Back and Pelvic Girdle Pain, Singapore 2016.

suggestions from scientific research – or from a completely different field – and would simply try something new.

This is why, four years on from its original publication, I felt personally impelled to revise this book based on the latest findings, because there was so much to add, rectify and expand upon. That was particularly important to me as my focus since 2016 has been specifically on research, and I now lead a new interdisciplinary research group at Ulm University. This highly specialised work is therefore always at the forefront of my mind – which is not necessarily the right approach for a book designed to be accessible to a more general readership. This is where I have to perform a balancing act between comprehensibility and clarity on the one hand, and scientific accuracy on the other, while also trying to avoid over-simplifying the content.

I would like to reassure my expert colleagues, who have been eagerly giving me their feedback on this book since 2014, that I am always on the side of science. At this level, I am always answerable to them. However, when it comes to writing a non-fiction book for a popular audience that's both interesting and easy to read – other linguistic rules apply, and I am quite happy to submit to them. In a scientific article, for example, if I were referring to an observed relationship – let's say, between age and mobility – I would also refer to what's known as the standard deviation, as well as citing several references from other literature. This simply isn't appropriate for a text designed for the general public, so we have dispensed with such scientific details in favour of readability. Having said that, this book is very much informed by the latest research, even if it isn't expressed with the same linguistic precision as I may use in a scientific publication. In this regard, I am happy to put my trust in the publisher and my co-author Johanna Bayer. After all, it is only by working together that we have succeeded in bringing our knowledge of how significant fascia is – for our bodies and our movements – into the broader consciousness, and keeping it there! Alongside my scientific work, that is one of my top priorities as a fascia researcher.

Robert Schleip
Ulm, Germany, November 2020

Introduction

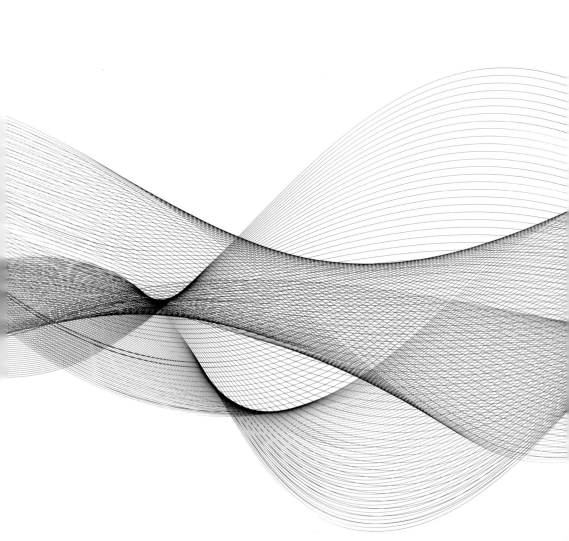

Why you need to exercise your fascia

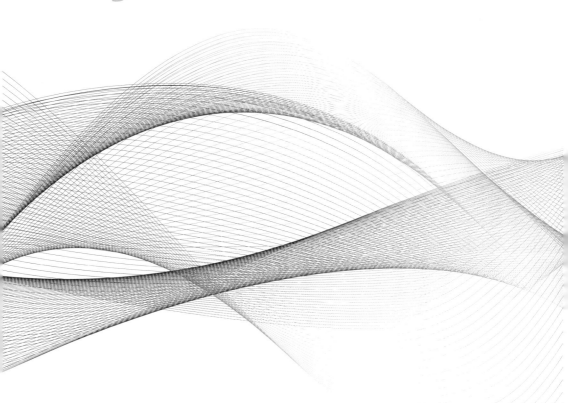

am fascinated by fascia. Fascia, more commonly known as connective tissue, is the soft tissue that runs through the entire body, surrounding our organs and giving us shape and structure. This material and its properties are so interesting that they took me on a journey from physical therapist to scientist. I wanted to know what role fascia plays in our physical movements and what it really means for the body and the mind. Throughout this journey, it became obvious to me that the importance of fascia cannot be overstated and that we would all benefit from becoming more aware of the influence that fascia has on our everyday lives, and especially on our athletic performance.

In this book, I will explain the significance and complexities of fascia, so that you can understand it too. Fascia has been on the sidelines for far too long, despite doctors, coaches and physiotherapists being well aware of its existence and functions. And yet in the past, when patients were suffering from chronic back pain requiring surgery, when physiotherapists wanted to alleviate pain and tension in their patients, or when athletes found their performance stagnating after many years of training,

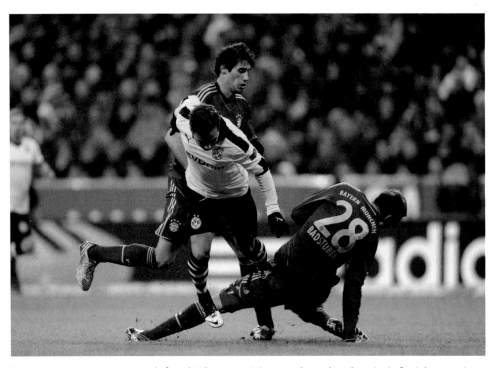

Sports injuries are most commonly found in ligaments, joint capsules and tendons, i.e. in fascial connective tissue. See how Holger Badstuber, who plays number 28 for Bayern Munich, tears the ligament in his right knee.

the focus was always on muscles, nerves, bones, coordination and strength. Fascia was never seen as a stand-alone cause. This has changed massively over the past few years, with fascia finally taking its place in the spotlight.

Many of the more recent findings relating to connective tissue have entirely discredited previous assumptions and – in some cases – caused a complete paradigm shift. Muscle soreness, for example, is not mainly due to the muscle tissue itself, but rather the fascia that surrounds the muscle. In many cases, back pain is caused by damage not to the vertebrae or intervertebral discs, but rather to the fascia. Sports injuries are, for the most part, not muscle problems, but fascial injuries. Fascia is now considered to be one of our most important sensory organs. The connective tissue even sends signals to the brain – the very heart of our consciousness. All our body movements are determined by sensors in fascia. If they fail, people can no longer control their movements.

The list of these new findings is enormous and is updated almost daily with information from all around the world. The information comes from various sources, including medical and biological research, physiotherapists and other practitioners. I worked as a body and movement therapist before I entered this field of science,

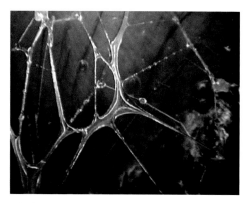

A hidden network: fascia. This unique microscopic image was taken by French surgeon J.C. Guimberteau.

so it is very important for me to connect theory and practice. In 2010, we at the Fascial Fitness Association had already begun to incorporate the many discoveries relating to fascia into a training program designed specifically to strengthen, stimulate and maintain the fascia. Today, the network of fascial researchers, sport scientists and kinesitherapists who use and develop this specific fascia training spans the entire globe.

There are already hundreds of books and training programs, all making more or less the same promises: increased energy, improved body strength, greater endurance, a more beautiful body, and better mobility, health and well-being. So if you're thinking, "What more could I possibly do?" – I completely understand. And if you're thinking, "Why should I switch to this training method? I'm doing fine as I am" – I understand that too. After all, as athletes well know, simply doing lots of training will not work – it has to be the right sort of training. And with fascia training, we're talking about something that, until recently, has been a complete unknown. However, focused fascia training can optimise your performance and allow you to achieve new personal bests. It also alleviates pain and stiffness in everyday life, and – above all – it is easy to incorporate into your existing training schedule. In other words, fascia training isn't there to replace all the previous training programs – it complements them. It enriches your training by adding in an element that has been missing until now. For many decades, the emphasis of sports science and training teachings has been on strength, stamina and coordination. The focus has therefore been on muscles, repetition and neural control, with no consideration for the fascia.

Many training programs claim that they do train the fascia, but this is only partly true. The programs are not efficient, as fascia requires its own impulses and specific movements. In common, fixed and stereotypical programs, these particular impulses are usually absent, or arise only coincidentally and not in a balanced quantity. In comparison, an athlete training for a marathon will inevitably also exercise their muscles. However, they will not be able to lift heavy weights, because their muscles have not been specifically developed for this task. Focused training is therefore the key to achieving optimum results.

Nowadays, we know about the enormous importance of fascia for ensuring the function and optimum coordination of our muscles, but we also know that fascia needs a special kind of stimulation. This knowledge is reflected in our training concepts, which have undergone several modifications over the years. Having previously focused on training individual muscles, the focus then turned to muscle groups and functional movements – and today a new approach is emerging. We now know that training should cover the entire fascial network and its long routes through the body. The condition of fascia influences how our injuries heal as well as our recovery after training and competition. It also determines much more – and this is what you will discover in this book.

So, you can view fascia training as the final piece in the jigsaw of your personal program. This doesn't mean that you need to do a ton of extra training or completely change your routine. The proposed exercises can be easily integrated into your current program and will seamlessly provide care and maintenance of the fascial network in your body. The exercises should stimulate the connective tissue, regenerate it, and keep it energised and supple, enabling you to train your muscles even more effectively, make your movements more fluid and elegant, and also increase your stamina. Because fascia training increases the capacity of the tendons and ligaments, it also avoids painful friction in hip joints and spinal discs, protects the muscles from injury, and keeps the body in shape, giving you a more youthful, toned physique. This is especially important for your day-to-day health, especially as you get older.

Fascia training is surprisingly easy: 10 minutes twice a week is plenty. There is no need for special clothing or equipment, and the entire program is simple and suitable for daily use and for all ages and levels of training. The advantages of fascia training for sport and in everyday life are simple:

▶ Your muscles work more efficiently.
▶ Recovery times are shorter, meaning you recuperate faster for the next workout and the next task.
▶ Your performance increases.
▶ Your movement and coordination improve.
▶ Your movements appear more elegant and less stiff.
▶ Your posture improves and your body appears more toned and youthful.
▶ The improved condition of your fascia provides long-term protection against pain and injury.

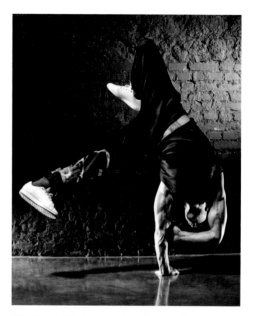

Whether it's hip hop, modern dance or ballet – what keeps dancers so strong and supple is having a well-trained and healthy fascia.

▶ You have more fun and variety in your training.
▶ Fascia training gives you a sense of youth and vitality.

The exercises in this book can also be adapted for different types of connective tissue or problem areas. Regular fascia training is also important with respect to ageing, which affects us all eventually. We're only as old as our connective tissue! Healthy fascia keeps you in shape and, with the right training, you can stay youthful and toned your whole life long. So if you want to stay young – or to feel young again – taking proper care of your fascia is a great place to start. As for everyday life, there are many positive effects to be enjoyed there too. Many of you will be familiar with the usual niggles that crop up time and again, sometimes going on to develop into even bigger problems. Whether it's back pain, shoulder and elbow problems, neck pain, tension, headaches and foot problems such as heel spurs, doctors are becoming increasingly aware that the condition of the connective tissue plays a key role in all these syndromes. It is now known that disorders in the connective tissue can even be the cause, for example, of shoulder problems such as the painful frozen shoulder, and that they can be treated with fascia-based treatments and exercise programs to alleviate or even eliminate the symptoms.

A journey into the undiscovered world of fascia

As a body therapist, researcher in human biology and teacher, I am acutely aware of fascia and its significance from a wide range of perspectives, both in my scientific work and in the training I provide to doctors, physiotherapists, Rolfing practitioners and osteopaths. But every day I also experience first-hand the role fascia plays in my own body: when I get up, enjoying a leisurely stretch in bed because it's such a soothing way to wake up; or when I clamber about on the climbing frame at the park around the corner from my house, stretching my joints to the maximum and making the local children laugh to see a man well into his 60s dangling from the monkey bars! Or first thing in the morning, when I jog barefoot to really feel my body and set my senses up for the day. Even when I'm at work where I spend a long time sitting at a desk, I do little exercises every so often to loosen up my rigid posture. There's no way I could cope with my current workload as a researcher, teacher and writer if I didn't take care of my body – and my fascial system in particular.

I hope that this book helps you to do the same, and to feel the benefit in your own body. I therefore invite you to join me on a journey into the previously undiscovered structures that literally make us who we are. We'll start by hunting for clues, and I'm afraid there will be a few areas to explore that are a little on the dry side, such as the chapters that explain the basics, including the anatomical and physiological details. However, they are simply part and parcel of learning the principles of fascia training, which go well beyond muscle training and strength building, delving deeply into the properties of the tissue. I firmly believe that gaining a deeper understanding into what's happening in the fascia not only has major benefits for athletes, coaches and exercise teachers, but also for more general readers who simply want to achieve a greater sense of body and movement.

This book has something for everyone, especially those experiencing pain, older people looking for a simple, practical training program and information, or complete novices who want a gentle way to become more active. This book has lots of practical tips, not only in the exercise chapter, but also in the section about nutrition and leading a healthy lifestyle.

On our journey into the undiscovered world of fascia, you will learn a lot of things that you may never have come across before. There will also be other things that you may have already encountered during your training or physiotherapy sessions. However, before we jump right in with the exercises, let's take a little time to get an overview of the properties and functions of fascia. This will help you to get so much more out of your training and even gain some new insights to take into your everyday life.

Above all else, our fascia training should be fun! In fact, sensory enjoyment is

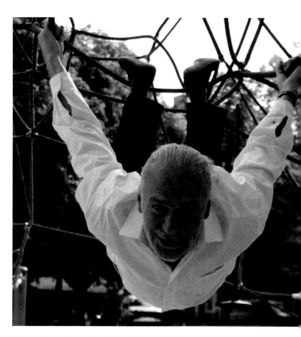

After a long day, there's nothing I find more rejuvenating than letting off some steam at the park near my apartment in Munich-Schwabing.

essential for our type of fascia training for a whole host of reasons – as you will find out later. So let's start our adventure by looking forward to gaining a new sense of joy in our own bodies and the way we move them.

Chapter 1

Fascia and connective tissue – what are they?

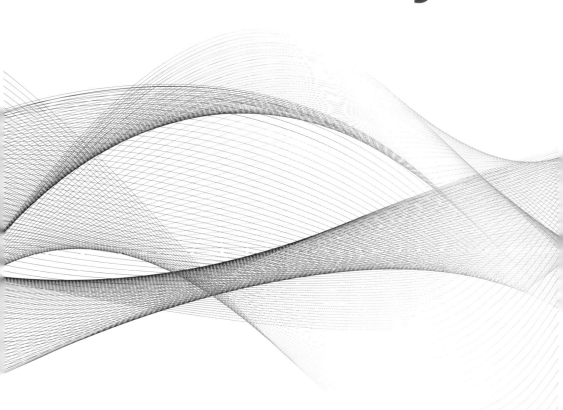

Before you start the exercises, it's time to learn more about fascia and the importance of the connective tissue in your body. The connective tissue is amazingly diverse and has features that affect the entire body. That's why I have dedicated this chapter to providing an overview of the different types of fascial tissue and their properties. As you will see, certain basic functions of the connective tissue are the same for almost all types. In addition, fascia is part of a network spanning long stretches of the body and is linked up with various organs. All this has implications for the type of training that my colleagues and I have developed, which will be introduced in Chapter 3. The attributes or features of connective tissue are even more important when you consider that they are related to pain, as well as to certain diseases or functional limitations, and that they change as we age and can even affect our mental health. For this reason, this chapter will also look more closely at the science of fascia.

If you want to get the most out of your workout, the following paragraphs are really important. Those of you who are in a hurry may wish to skip this chapter and head straight to the exercises in Chapter 3. In a quiet moment, however, you should come back and read this information, as you will benefit even more when doing the exercises and perhaps gain some insights into ways of adapting your daily routine, too.

Fresh fascia

At some time or another, most people will probably have had a piece of fascial tissue in their hand, usually in the kitchen while cutting meat. When we prepare meat, it is usually taken from the muscle of the animal, and that is usually where we find fascia. It runs through the pieces of meat, creating a delicate marbling effect, and also appears as a white layer on top of the meat. Butchers, chefs and home cooks tend to cut off the tendons and almost all of the white layers. Depending on the type of meat and the dish being prepared, they are sometimes kept in to add flavour and richness. If, for example, you like nice crispy crackling on your roast pork, then you would leave a thick piece of abdominal fascia, including fat, on the joint. In a typical roast beef joint that is cut from the loin, you can see part of the large fascia found in the animal's back, as shown in the picture. It has been scored, ready for roasting. The fascia that you can see here is muscular fascia, but there are also other types of fascial tissue, such as that found in the intestines. However, the focus of this book is the musculoskeletal system, so we will be looking mainly at the muscle fascia.

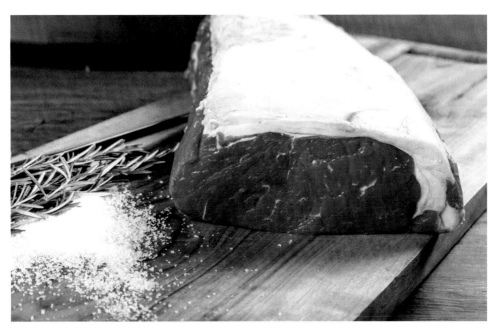

Fascia up close: typical roast beef joint, with a fine marbling of fat and connective tissue. The white layer on top is a section of the large fascia found in the back.

The basic building block with many functions

Fascia is essentially made up of the two core building blocks of any living organism: protein and water. The exact structure of the tissue depends on the function it serves and its location in the body. There is so much variation in the different types of fascia and their many functions that it can all be very confusing to understand. Until recently, even the experts were divided in their understanding of fascia. However, doctors, physiologists and anatomists have long been aware that the large sheets of fascia, as well as the tendons and ligaments, the firm sheaths of tissue encasing our organs – such as the heart and kidneys – and the ultra-thin layers around the bundles of muscle and joint capsules are all made of the same material. They are also in agreement that all the subcutaneous fat, the loose, reticulate abdominal tissue, and even the cartilage and fatty tissue all share the same essential principles when it comes to structure and function. In fact, all the connective tissue acts as a kind of universal building material within the body. It is all part of a mesh of fibres that are tightly bound in some places and looser in others, and contain varying amounts of fluid. This mesh can be stretchy or dense, resistant to tension and tearing or very soft and loose, but it always consists of the same core building blocks – just in different proportions: collagen, elastin and a watery to gel-like ground substance.

At the first International Fascia Research Congress in 2007, the founders, including myself, decided to redefine the term. The fibrous connective tissue in the musculoskeletal system and the solid sheaths of tissue around the organs was henceforth known as 'fascia'. We wanted a term that also accounted for the fact that the connective tissue has various functions in common. In coming up with the term, our event team drew upon the findings that had been made by doctors, physiologists, biologists, orthopaedic surgeons and anatomists, as well as physiotherapists and massage therapists, movement therapists and alternative therapists from all disciplines since the 1960s.

When this book was first published in 2014, there was still some criticism from the medical world about our use of the word 'fascia' as a comprehensive term for this tissue. However, that has all changed since then, with the concept of an interdependent network of fascia in the human body having now been widely accepted by orthopaedic surgeons and sports scientists. Fascia training has also received a certain amount of criticism, with some claiming that "you cannot exercise the fascia specifically because it is inseparable from the muscles."

This statement, which does seem plausible at first glance, has been put forward time and again, including by some highly regarded experts in the field. However, this is also something that my colleagues have since come to understand differently. It is becoming increasingly recognised that the collagen tissue we call fascia has different sensitivity thresholds and adjustment times than the muscle fibres, and that it therefore makes perfect sense to practice targeted exercises that hone in on the fascia. In some instances, those very same critics who were vehemently opposed to the notion of being able to exercise the fascia independently when we published the first edition of the book have – to our sheer delight – made a complete U-turn and are now passionate advocates of fascia training.

The components of fascia

Collagens

Collagens play a very important role as a component of fascia. They consist of fairly densely-packed fibres that literally give the human body – and that of all vertebrates – its shape. They are therefore referred to as scaffold proteins or structural proteins. Making up a proportion of

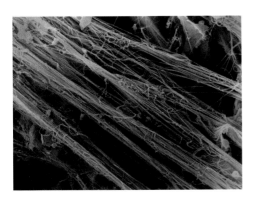

These images of collagen fibres were taken using a scanning electron microscope with extreme magnification.

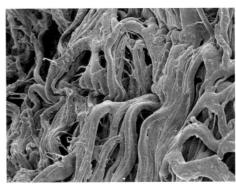

A significantly enlarged image of elastin fibres from the main artery.

30 percent, collagens are the most common proteins in the body, so they really are one of our core building blocks. Even bones are originally made from collagen fibres. In the womb, the embryo initially produces collagen. Then minerals, such as calcium, are incorporated between the collagen layers. This is how hard bones develop from soft fibres.

There are 28 different types of collagen, four of which are very common. They have some interesting mechanical characteristics: they stretch easily while also being very resistant to tearing, and their tensile strength is greater than that of steel!

Elastin

Elastin is the second most-common structural protein found in fascial tissue. Elastin fibres are particularly stretchy: when pulled, they can expand by up to 150 percent of their original length and then return to their previous shape, like an elastic band. The name 'elastin' refers to this important property, because elastin can expand to more than double its length before tearing due to too much strain.

This stretchiness is important for organs that are subjected to mechanical stress or that have to change their shape – such as the bladder, which perpetually fills and empties. Thanks to their high proportion of elastin, these organs can extend and contract again like a balloon. Our skin, which stretches naturally when we move, also contains elastin.

However, it is not the elastin fibres that are responsible for the elasticity of fascia. Elastin is indeed very stretchy, like chewing gum, but it is the collagen fibres that store kinetic energy and release it again, allowing it to spring back like a cat-apult. We will explain this phenomenon in more detail in the next chapter. For now, the important thing to grasp is the difference between elastin and collagen fibres. The confusion lies in our everyday language: when we talk about 'elasticity', it is often unclear whether we are refer-ring to the property of being very stretchy, like chewing gum, or having a high stor-age capacity for kinetic energy, like a steel spring. Elastin fibres are characterised by the former property, while collagen fibres possess the latter.

Connective tissue cells

Both of the fibrous proteins collagen and elastin are produced by cells in fas-cia – the actual connective tissue. These cells are called fibroblasts and are spread throughout the mesh of fibres that make up the fascial tissue. Only the fibroblasts produce the connective tissue fibres in the amount needed by the correspond-ing organ. They also respond to external requirements. For example, if you work out a lot and develop strength, the fibro-blasts make more fibres that help your muscles to grow. These connective tis-sue cells also regularly regenerate the tis-sue, but this is a very slow process. It takes you more than six months to renew most of your collagen fibres. In fact, it usually takes 7 to 14 months for the old material to be broken down and replaced with new fibres.

As well as producing the structural pro-teins your body needs, the connective tissue cells also produce enzymes and neurotransmitters, which enable the fibro-blasts to communicate with one another and with other cells. With these neuro-transmitters, they are also involved in the functioning of the immune system. These biochemical elements, together with the watery to gel-like fluid in which they float, are referred to by specialists as 'ground substance'.

The matrix

The connective tissue cells and fibres are surrounded by fluid in which other sub-stances float. This mixture of fibres and ground substance is called the 'matrix'. The fluid element of the ground sub-stance consists of water and sugar mol-ecules, whose job it is to bind various materials and cells together.

The matrix plays a crucial role in sup-plying nutrients to the connective tis-sue cells, and to the organ to which the connective tissue belongs. We will revisit this subject later on, when the deeper secrets of fascia will be discussed from a scientific perspective. It is important to note that the matrix in these different connective tissue types hosts large quan-tities of immune cells, lymphocytes or fat cells, nerve endings and blood vessels, and that the water content of the matrix varies.

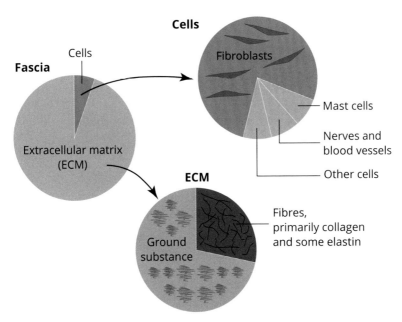

The structure of fascia: the ratio of the components, the exact composition and the type of fibres depend on what function the fascia has within the body and on the organ to which the tissue belongs.

Water is crucial as a medium for cellular metabolism. As a consequence, the various techniques used to treat fascia focus on the water content and on the exchange of fluid – which we will come to later. There is another very important component of the matrix that is also responsible for its water content: a substance known as hyaluronan, previously called 'hyaluronic acid', within the beauty industry, for example. Experts recently agreed on this new name, partly because it is not actually an acid. Chemically, hyaluronan is a sugar molecule. Hyaluronan is produced by special connective tissue cells known as fasciacytes, and can change its consistency from a thick gel to a watery lubricant. It therefore forms the synovial fluid – the

substance that lubricates the joints in our knees, shoulders and hips, for example. Because hyaluronan is so effective at storing water, it also plays an important role in the proportion of fluid in the loose types of connective tissue. There are also high levels of this substance found in the spinal discs. Hyaluronan stores a lot of water between the collagen and elastin fibres in the skin, which is what gives faces that much sought-after plump, wrinkle-free complexion. That is why the substance is so popular in the cosmetics industry. Hyaluronan is commonly used in creams and other preparations, and it has become a very popular treatment for plumping the lips of celebrities and non-celebrities alike.

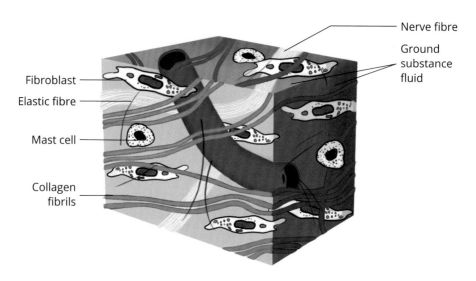

Nerve fibre

Ground substance fluid

Fibroblast

Elastic fibre

Mast cell

Collagen fibrils

Loose connective tissue has many components. This image depicts a cross-section of tissue.

Types and functions of connective tissue

The astonishing ubiquity of fascia in the body reflects the diversity of its types and functions. They can be loosely categorised into the following types of tissue:

Loose, fibrous connective tissue

Fibrous connective tissue contains quite a lot of ground substance, specifically fluid, but also connective tissue cells, as well as collagen and elastin fibres. It is knotted in the form of a soft, coarse mesh. Gaps in the abdomen around the organs are filled with loose connective tissue which protects, stabilises and cushions the organs. The connective tissue also has very important functions for the metabolism and supplying nutrients to the internal organs. Loose connective tissue plumps our skin in the lower layers and accommodates hair follicles, sebaceous and sweat glands, blood vessels and many nerve endings, as well as sensors receptive to pressure, touch, movement or temperature. Typical of loose connective tissue is its wealth of immune and lymphatic cells, as well as the fact that, like the skin, it contains many nerve endings, motion receptors, glands and other cells. This type of tissue forms the highest proportion of connective tissue in the body.

Elastic connective tissue

Elastic connective tissue contains a high proportion of elastin. This type of tissue can be found in organs that are subjected to more intense stretching, such as the dermis, bladder, gall bladder, aorta and the lungs.

Parallel, tight, fibrous connective tissue

Parallel connective tissue, with its very high proportion of collagen, forms the tendons, the ligaments, the solid capsules around the organs (such as the kidneys) and the pericardium, as well as all the thin layers of fascia surrounding the muscles. The fibres are aligned parallel to each other, pointing in the direction in which stress usually occurs, for either anatomical or physiological reasons. Their parallel arrangement enables them to resist very strong tensile forces.

Irregular connective tissue

There is less ground substance and very little elastin in irregular connective tissue. By contrast, it is densely packed with fibres, especially thick collagen bundles. This sort of tissue is what forms the lining of the brain and the subcutaneous tissue or dermis. It is able to withstand high levels of pressure and tensile strain. Its fibres run in various directions, allowing it to move with the different tensile forces to which it is subjected. Because it can be pulled in several directions, it is referred to within the medical profession as 'multi-directional' tissue. The connective tissue cells are typically squeezed in between the fibres, and it has a significantly lower fluid content than in loose connective tissue – although it is still over 60 percent.

The grapefruit principle: fascia holds everything in shape

Info

All of our internal organs are literally surrounded by fascia. It permeates our entire bodies, in various surface layers as well as in the deeper layers. A colleague of mine, Thomas Myers, uses this vivid image of a grapefruit to illustrate the way that fascia holds the entire body in shape. The pulp of the grapefruit is enclosed in small detachments of white skin, and on the outside it is again surrounded by a solid white skin that fits snugly to the peel.

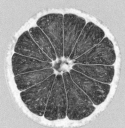

If you were to remove all the pulp and leave only the white skin, you could reconstruct the entire fruit and its shape on the basis of this structure alone. The same principle applies to fascia and its function in the human body. It is possible to see how a person looks based solely on the connective tissue, without the flesh and bones. The same does not apply, however, to the skeleton.

Reticular connective tissue

Reticular connective tissue consists of a type of collagen that can form very thin fibres. It is typical of the connective tissue of the spleen, lymph nodes and thymus gland, and is commonly found on freshly healing scars.

> ### The connective tissue: facts and figures
>
> Each person has, on average, between 18 and 23 kg of connective tissue. This tissue:
>
> ▶ Stores a quarter of the total amount of water in the body.
> ▶ Provides cells and organs with nutrients.
> ▶ Responds to stress and strain, and adapts accordingly.
> ▶ Continuously regenerates itself, albeit slowly. It usually takes between 7 and 14 months for collagen fibres to be replaced.
> ▶ Increasingly loses water as we age.
> ▶ Becomes matted with age and inactivity.

Special connective tissue

Adipose or fatty tissue, cartilage and the gelatinous substance of the umbilical cord are also types of connective tissue. However, adipose or fatty tissue contains less ground substance and less collagen. It is made up of specialised cells known as adipocytes, which store fat rather than water. These fat cells are surrounded by elastin fibres. Fat has a surprising number of functions in the body: it stores energy, insulates against cold, secretes hormones and neurotransmitters, is very metabolically active, cushions organs (e.g. the kidneys) and joints (e.g. the knees and heels), and forms typical parts of the body, such as the thighs, buttocks or breasts.

A new way of looking at the body

As I write, anatomists and other fascia researchers around the world, such as Carla Stecco from the University of Padua and Hanno Steinke at the University of Leipzig, are working on new ways of representing the human body, particularly in regard to fascia. The *Functional Atlas of the Human Fascial System* by Carla Stecco, which was published in 2016, contains innovative representations by her and other researchers that is revolutionising our understanding of fascia. Among other things, Stecco illustrates how the first tough layer of fascial tissue beneath the skin surrounds almost the entire body like a wetsuit.

The four basic functions of fascia

The list of different connective tissue types might appear confusing at first, but they divide quite simply into four basic functions:

► **Shape:** to encase, cushion, protect and give structure.
► **Movement:** to transfer and store energy, maintain tension and stretch.
► **Supply:** to metabolise energy, transport fluid and carry nutrients.
► **Communication:** to receive and transmit stimuli and information.

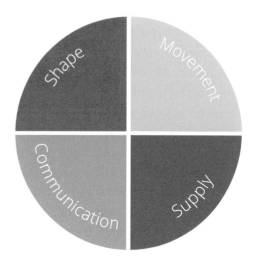

A continuum with four dimensions: the basic functions of fascia. Fascia performs various functions throughout the entire body.

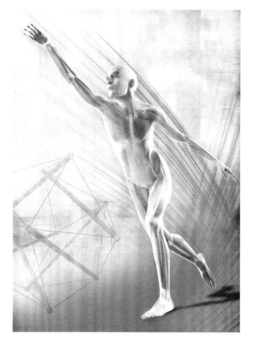

White instead of red: this is how the latest anatomical representations show how our body looks beneath the skin.

Since the various functions almost always occur together, complement each other, and are mutually dependent, they are seen as a kind of continuum. That is why they are represented by a circle – you will see this symbol a lot as you work your way through the book.

The four basic functions are therefore associated with each type of fascia or connective tissue, no matter which body part or organ it serves. Only the proportions and priorities shift: some parts of the muscle fibres contain more water and serve as suppliers, while others have less water. The tendons, for example, have virtually no functionality as suppliers. All fascial tissue, however, sends signals (it contains receptors and sensors), and also supports body movement.

Shaping and movement are based purely on the mechanical properties of the material. Fascia performs mechanical and static functions within the body. It gives us shape and structure, enables us to tense our muscles and move our limbs, as well as providing support and protection and encasing or padding out parts of the body. Anatomists were aware of these functions as far back as the Middle Ages. However, for a long time they assigned the responsibility of actions mainly to the muscles, bones and other organs, while the connective tissue was seen as passive or even dead, in a similar sense to the hair and nails.

Nowadays we know that not to be true, because the tissue almost always performs the two other basic functions as well – those of supply and communication. These are physiological actions that can only be performed by living tissue. Moreover, the fact that every organ in the body is surrounded by fascia makes it indispensable for the whole process of cell metabolism, for our inner perception of movement and organ activity, and for the transmission of many signals throughout the body.

The medical profession has had a basic awareness of the physiological functions of the fascial network since the end of the 19th century. However, it has only been in recent years, since around the 1960s, that these functions have been systematically explored. Since then, our understanding of the connective tissue has changed dramatically, from the early perception of it as dead tissue there only to provide shape and support, to its recognition as an organ in its own right – and even as an indispensable sensory organ.

Of particular importance are the physiological functions of the connective tissue around the organs and under the skin. This tissue facilitates the metabolism of cells and organs, and is a medium through which lymphs, blood vessels and nerves can run, as well as accommodating water and nutrient exchange and containing many immune cells. Physiologists nowadays consider the general metabolic function of the connective tissue as its central role within the body. And since the loose connective tissue under the skin runs like a network throughout our body, researchers have come to see it as a communication phenomenon: if the supply network is disturbed or damaged at any point, the reactions and stress responses within the connective tissue will span the entire body.

There will be a section later in the book where we will look more closely at the science of fascia. You will also read more about the four basic functions in the discussion of the four dimensions of fascia training in Chapter 2.

Severing ties with invasive surgery

Werner Klingler, with whom I worked in fascial research at the University of Ulm, is a senior physician in anaesthesiology. He spends almost every day in the operating room, which resembles a high-tech workshop, with advanced endoscopes and many monitors on which doctors can observe processes inside the body during surgery. He knows from his older colleagues that surgery was once an extremely daunting and invasive ordeal. In order to access the organs in the abdominal cavity during an operation – the gall bladder or the appendix, for example – they had to make long and deep incisions. To do this, the fibrous pad of connective tissue would be moved aside, severed, or even cut away entirely. This was done out of necessity – surgeons simply wanted to get to the site of the problem in order to work there as efficiently as possible. The unremarkable-looking tissue was thought only to play a subordinate role. The organs would therefore be exposed and operated on, after which the surgeon would sew up the abdominal wall, often taking pride in their beautiful stitching. Surgeons recognised that, by doing this, they were damaging sensitive internal tissue and causing scars and adhesions that would permanently affect the organ and its supply – but there was no other solution.

Only gradually, thanks to the advances of technology, has it been discovered that it is far better for patients to have smaller scars and the least possible injury to the internal abdominal cavity (even if it is 'only' the padding tissue that is affected). Keeping as much of the connective tissue intact as possible meant they experienced less pain, the wounds healed faster, and there was less damage and fewer post-surgical complications. This was so self-evident that a set of special procedures was developed, which is now known as keyhole surgery. This entails operations using small cameras, optical instruments and micro-surgical devices, which allow smaller openings to be made in the skin and the body. Surgeons refer to these procedures as minimally invasive. Keyhole surgery leaves only very small incisions and interventions, particularly in the inner tissue. Many studies have confirmed that, when there are fewer cuts in the connective tissue and less scarring, the wound heals better, the patients experience less pain and the recovery period is shorter.

The whole thing stemmed from a common error – and one that not only sports medics had fallen foul of. It simply was not taken into account how closely connected the fascia in the intestines is to the fascia in the musculoskeletal system. This unhelpful separation was in part due to the lack of communication between different medical disciplines. We now know that disturbances in the intestinal fascia can lead to significant postural disorders and vice versa. In addition, vessels and nerves have their own fascial sheaths, such as the sciatic nerve that runs down the back of the leg and is about as thick as a finger, or the bundles of vascular nerves that radiate from the neck into the arms. Surgery can cause scars and matting of the fascial tissue, which can interfere with its ability to glide smoothly beneath the skin. This can result in pain and restricted movement even in parts of the body that are nowhere near the surgical site.

Despite the new techniques, however, surgeons still have some way to go. As has been shown, minimally invasive procedures leave smaller scars on the skin, which cause fewer cosmetic implications. This is appealing to patients – after all, who wants to have a big scar on their stomach? However, it also means that surgeons have to try to find more and more inconspicuous entry points, which are often far away from the site of surgery. Depending on how the target organ is accessed, the surgeon still has to cut through fascial tissue – sometimes to an even greater extent than in the past, when the incision would be made directly above the organ. In an effort to make the incision in the most unobtrusive location, the cut the surgeon has to make may even be bigger than it would have been before. As a result, whole layers of fascia now become

severed, over long stretches of tissue, and incisions and injuries pass horizontally through the connective tissue, whereas in the past the procedure would have been to make a vertical cut. As I am sure you can gather, the new approach is not without its problems. It has become even clearer that surgery has to be executed as carefully as possible because of the connective tissue, but there is still no universal method indicating how best to achieve this. One of several approaches, for example, is to spread the adjoined layers of fascia apart using blunt scissors, rather than cutting through them with a sharp blade.

High performance: fascia and the musculoskeletal system

The connective tissues in the musculoskeletal system are what allow our bodies to perform, mechanically and physiologically, at such a high level. The fact that we can move at all is largely down to the fascia. Each individual muscle, each individual bundle of fibres and even each individual fibre itself is surrounded by thin layers of fascia. These sheaths transfer the force of the muscle fibres, allow the bundles of fibres to glide smoothly, and reduce friction between the muscle and any adjacent tissue so that they can function properly. The tight fascial tissue known as

The power couple: muscle and fascia

Info

Muscles are composed of many thousands of fibres packed into tight bundles. Each bundle is wrapped in a thin layer of fascial tissue. This whole structure is again enclosed in an outer muscle fascia, which ensures that the muscle retains its shape.

Muscle fibres: Muscles consist of thousands of fibrous structures.
Endomysium: This razor-thin fascial sheath surrounds individual muscle fibres.
Fibre bundles: Thousands of fibres form dense bundles.
Perimysium: The fibre bundles are each surrounded by connective tissue.
Epimysium: The outermost fascial sheath of muscle maintains the muscle's shape.

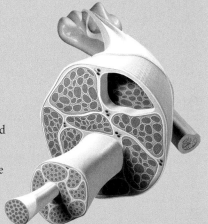

Connective tissue sheaths in a piece of lean meat seen under the microscope. Japanese researchers dissolved red muscle tissue in caustic soda, so that just the honeycombed sheaths remain. Top left is the epimysium; top right is the endomysium, which encases a single muscle fibre. The lower image shows a cross-section through the inside of a muscle. In addition to the abundance of

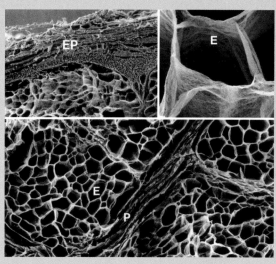

endomysia (E), you can see the perimysium (P), which encases the different bundles of muscle fibre and also separates them from each other.

the tendon transfers the energy from the muscle to the bone. Tendons and tendon sheaths therefore also belong to the fascial structure of the muscle. Every muscle is connected by tendons to bone attachment points. In addition, long interconnections of fascial muscle units link up several body parts to each other. This occurs over long distances in our body – from the feet, over the back and all the way to the head, or along the sides of the body.

Dissected and ignored

For decades, the fascia around the muscles suffered the same fate as the fascia found in the abdominal cavity, with these inconspicuous layers of connective tissue being largely ignored by medical science. Instead, the focus of anatomists was diverted to the eye-catching lean red flesh and its visible function under the skin. On their dissecting tables, they neatly peeled back all the white stuff from the skin and muscles – the connective tissue – and pulled the red flesh free to describe its form and function. Of course, they knew and saw that all the muscles were completely wrapped in and permeated by connective tissue. At best, however, the professionals paid attention to the thick tendons, ligaments, and flat fascia that visibly connects the muscles to the bone. The consequences of this are well known: even today, anatomical illustrations and studies of musculoskeletal systems essentially show the skeleton and muscles. Anatomical atlases are full of parcels of red muscle – the associated connective tissue simply doesn't feature. Only a few major sheets of fascia are visible, which are regarded as distribution centres, such as the large fascia found in the back. Even the major works of anatomy only devote a few pages to connective tissue.

Incidentally, a crucial element is situated right next to the bone: a fibrous tissue layer, or what doctors refer to as the 'periosteum'. The bones, like all organs of the body, are wrapped in a layer of connective tissue. Think of the image of the grapefruit we saw earlier: everything is encased. The tendons, therefore, are not

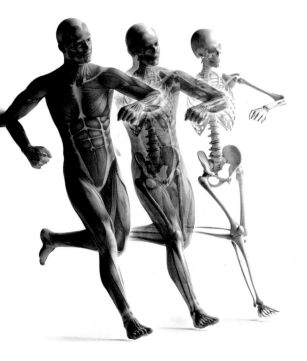

Muscles and bones, but barely any fascia in sight: a typical anatomical study of human movement, with the connective tissue missing.

usually attached to the hard bone itself, but to its outer skin – the periosteum.

The muscles themselves, even the smallest of them, contain elastic fibres that are specially designed to withstand tensile stress. They also contain structural proteins called actin and titin, which give the motor cells their mobility. Actin is found in the cell membrane of the muscle cell itself and enables the cell to move. Titin supports the muscle fibre by returning it to its starting position after a contraction. It is similar to collagen and elastin, but has a much longer structure. Like actin, it is specifically a component of the muscle rather than the connective tissue. Its function within the muscle is two-fold: internally, the elasticity of the fibres enable the muscle cells to contract; while externally, it creates the shape of the muscle.

Information centres: fascia as a sensory organ

Inside the small, fine layers and thicker layers of fascial tissue in and around the muscles, there run all the vital nerves and blood vessels that supply the muscle. An abundance of receptors send and receive information to and from the muscle and forward this information to the brain. These receptors are nerve endings of various types; they derive their information from deeper in the central nervous system and communicate details about stretching, movement, the position of the muscle in question, the organ and the body part. The individual nerve endings are known as:

▸ Pacinian corpuscles
▸ Ruffini corpuscles
▸ Golgi receptors, and
▸ interstitial receptors.

Medically speaking, all four types belong to the category of 'mechanoreceptors'. These are sensors that register motion, changes in position, pressure, touch or stretching. They specialise in different qualities of stimulus and intensity.

Pacinian corpuscles react to rapid pressure changes, vibrations or to jerky impulses. These particles require alternations in motion or impulse. If the force does not change over a longer period of time, they will cease to respond.

Ruffini corpuscles are programed to respond to gradual changes in pressure. They therefore react to more steady stimuli, such as relaxation massage or slow stretching at the gym.

Golgi receptors do not respond to passive stimuli, but instead to muscle activity. To put it more precisely, they respond to the tensile stress on the muscle caused by the tendon, but only above a certain strength. These receptors are situated in the tissue where the tendon meets the muscle. When the tendon pulls on the muscle with enough force to cause a contraction, the Golgi receptors reduce the muscle tension. In this way, they protect the tendons and the joints from being overloaded.

Interstitial receptors are connected to the autonomic nervous system, which controls unconscious processes and movements, such as digestion and blood pressure. In addition to pressure, they signal pain and temperature. They are also the most common type of receptor.

All four types of receptor contribute to the innate ability we call 'proprioception', our internal self-perception of the spatial position and movement of our bodies. The fact that such proprioceptive sensors exist, especially in the deeper layers of connective tissue of the skin and the joints, is by no means newly acquired knowledge. Even in the past, this seemed logical, as the skin is a major touch organ and is stretched in a multitude of ways, and because the joints are moved so often. Physiologists and neurologists were therefore unsurprised by the existence of stimulus detectors. What is new, however, is that these sensors also colonise the muscular fascia and the tendons, constantly sending signals to the brain. Amazingly, they appear in far greater numbers even than the nerve fibres that

cause muscle movement, namely motor neurons: nerves such as the sciatic nerve consist of almost three times as many sensory neurons as motor neurons. Therefore, human movements seem to depend mainly on the sense of movement initiated through the nervous system, rather than triggered muscular activity.

As physiologists only recently found out, the number of different sensors and nerve endings in the fascia around the muscle far exceeds the number in the muscle itself. This is especially true for those who report pain, as pain arises primarily in the fascia and not in the muscle. We will look at this profound phenomenon in more detail later on. Several years ago, it was discovered that the deep fascia spanning the back is covered with pain sensors. This shed new light on the chronic, unexplained back pain from which so many people suffer.

A direct line to the nervous system

These new discoveries in physiology have completely changed the way we look at connective tissue: specifically, the fascia of the musculoskeletal system is now considered a sensory organ in its own right – a prolific internal information system that is essential for brain functioning. Because our brain seems to rely on these continuous stimuli, it has almost come to expect the wealth of information that it constantly receives from fascia. The self-perception of the body is of fundamental importance, even for seemingly simple activities such as standing upright. This sense of our own movements is often called the 'sixth sense', but it is more technically known as depth perception, motion perception or proprioception.

This inner awareness comes from the fascia around our organs, because it contains the nerve endings, receptors and sensors that deliver all the various pieces of information: the position and location of the organs within the space, their actions and movements, pressure and touch, temperature, and even their biochemical make-up. In this respect, fascia can almost be seen as part of the brain and the nervous system, which controls movement.

The connection of the fascial sensors to the autonomic nervous system – previ-ously known as the vegetative nervous system – is just as interesting. It explains, for example, why treating fascia with massage or manual therapy has certain effects which cannot be merely due to the mechanical pressure applied by the hands, such as the sense of heaviness or lightness in a certain body part, warmth, a feeling of relaxation in the muscle, reduced blood pressure, increased or lowered heart rate, or even bowel movements. These activities are regulated by the autonomic nervous system. Therefore, if they occur, it has to be because the autonomic nervous system has been activated. This would suggest that treatments using the hands, such as pressure and massage, activate the motion sensors in the fascial tissue; in particular the Ruffini corpuscles and the interstitial receptors. These sensors send signals to the spinal cord, which in turn changes the muscle tension or the stress state of the blood

The importance of fascia

▶ Muscles would not be able to function or keep their shape without their fascial sheaths – they would simply spill out like thick treacle.

▶ The number of sensors in fascia far exceeds the number of sensors in the muscles.

▶ Fascia reports information about movement, position, tension, pressure and pain to the brain and autonomic nervous system.

▶ In terms of area, fascia is our largest sensory organ – even larger than the skin.

▶ Fascia is crucial to our perception of our own body.

An unusual case

Ian Waterman – the man who couldn't feel his body

There are a few rare neurological diseases which specifically cause the patient to lose their sense of proprioception. These patients – of which there are very few in the world – are not paralysed as such, yet they are unable to move normally because they have lost their 'sixth sense', i.e. their sense of movement.

This loss of perception is usually caused by a viral infection, which leads to false responses within the immune system. The immune system is derailed and therefore goes into attack, destroying specifically those nerve pathways that inform the brain about what the muscles, tendons, ligaments and joints are doing. This causes the patient to lose all sense of movement within the body – something that is normally processed constantly by the brain on an unconscious level. However, the ability to sense pain, cold and heat all remain intact. The motor neurons are not affected either, meaning that, in principle, the patient can still move their body. The muscles can still be controlled, in that patients can tense all their muscles while sitting in a wheelchair, for example. However, they are unable to stand up or walk independently. Standing and walking are complex tasks requiring intense coordination, but the brain is unable to receive the required information from the nerve endings in fascia. It is the fascia, therefore, that communicates the loss of proprioception. Taking this disease as a starting point, neurologists have finally been able to gauge the significance of this 'sixth sense' for the automatic control of movement.

Ian Waterman from the UK suffers from the loss of proprioception, and has a vehement determination to overcome it. Since becoming impaired by the illness, he has been training himself to move his body consciously – and it does work, albeit with a great deal of effort. Ian has to consciously trigger and control every movement his body makes, rather than just letting them happen automatically. This is all about vision. If Ian were standing in a lit room and the light was switched off, he would fall to the ground because his conscious control fails when he cannot see anything: his body no longer has an organ to control his movements internally. I had the pleasure of meeting him in person as part of a scientific study, and was incredibly impressed by his wilful determination to beat his motion blindness. While walking and moving happen mostly unconsciously for a healthy person, for Ian, it's like running a marathon every day. Of all known cases of the condition, he is also the only individual who has managed to walk again independently. He is a tour de force.

The BBC made a documentary about Ian Waterman's story that is well worth a watch. It is called 'The Man Who Lost his Body' and you should be able to find it online.

vessels. It therefore has to be the case that fascia and the signals it transmits to the nervous system and the brain are what is behind the responses that physical therapists and physicians have long been aware of, but for which they had no concrete explanation in terms of the origin or mode of action (see Chapter 4).

The science of fascia

The many findings that have been accumulated by fascia researchers the world over are as yet unclear in terms of their scope. One thing for certain is that they have changed the opinion of doctors concerning numerous disease patterns. They also present some brand-new perspectives with regard to anatomy, sports science and kinesiology, the regulation of bodily functions, phenomena such as scarring

and wound healing, and even mental health and brain function.

Of course, modern fascia researchers did not start from scratch. Knowledge about the role of the connective tissue has been around since the 19th century, and pioneers have since made some ground-breaking discoveries. Some of those pioneers were established professors such as Alfred Pischinger, while others were scientists such as the biochemist Ida P. Rolf. However, there has also been great progress made by physiotherapists like Elisabeth Dicke or autodidacts with no formal medical training such as Andrew Taylor Still, the founder of osteopathy. They all stressed the importance of connective tissue, physical movement and manual therapy – aspects that we now have the means to investigate on a more scientific level.

Fascial pioneers

Alfred Pischinger and his system of basic regulation

Alfred Pischinger (1899–1983) was an Austrian histologist and embryologist who taught as a professor of medicine at the University of Graz and later in Vienna, where he also carried out medical research.

Alfred Pischinger depicted the human body as a self-regulating and networked system, in which information about different subsystems is passed on and processed. In his view, the connective tissue had a key role as an intermediary, affecting vital basic functions such as blood pressure and immune defence. He referred to this role as 'basic regulation', and described treatments based on this tissue as holistic because they take into account the cross-linked nature of the body.

Pischinger's image of cells and their metabolism was that of a friendly environment, which the cell needs in the same way that a unicellular organism needs seawater. This environment allows the cell to obtain nutrients, disposes of metabolites and exchanges signals. The way the cell communicates with its environment is a two-way relationship. All the surrounding cells are dependent on this environment – the matrix.

As early as 1933, Austrian-born Pischinger became a member of the Nazi party. He was a supporting member of the SS and later, while at the University of Graz, he became a leading member of a group of Nazi doctors who dealt with eugenics. His Nazi past unfortunately casts a huge shadow over his professional accomplishments. After the war and denazification, Pischinger became a professor in Vienna, where he was highly honoured for his research into physiology. He died there in 1983.

From therapist to researcher

My personal interest in fascia was first sparked by my practical work in the field. In the 1980s, I set up my own Rolfing clinic in Munich, which I found so interesting that I gave up my other profession as a psychologist. Working with the human body in a physical sense was so much more exciting to me.

In 1988, I became more engaged with the theories behind Rolfing. That said, I also began to question those theories. Some of the teachings seemed fairly questionable, and I was no longer as convinced by the ideas of our pioneer, Ida P. Rolf. According to Rolf theory, fascia is made up of solid collagen fibres that create a physical frame. As such, our role as therapists is to continually form and deform this frame with our hands like clay or plasticine. This is not in line with my own experiences as a manual therapist, although I did know that I was definitely causing something to happen: the tissue, muscles and posture of my patients literally changed in my hands. Yet this occurred not only due to the intense pressure I was applying, but often also as a result of the flowing, slow, melting movements used in Rolfing therapy.

I just knew that there had to be other mechanisms at play. Further explanations were thrown into the mix – the usual eso-

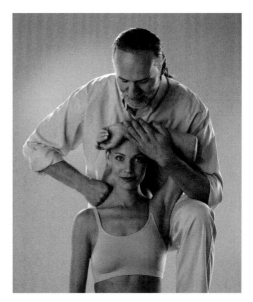

My first experiences working with fascia came about through my career as a Rolfing practitioner.

teric trends like energy flow, meridians and blockages, for example – but none of these interpretations were satisfactory. I wanted to look at the other point of view – the scientific aspect. Ida Rolf herself was a biochemist, and in my psychology studies in Heidelberg I had learned a bit about the basic principles of scientific thinking and serious scientific research, medical and psychological methods in statistics, the biological context, the nervous system and the main body functions. I thought that if we therapists were proving that Rolfing and manual therapy works, then it must be possible to find examples – in the form of traceable, measurable processes – of these mechanisms at work within the body.

Fascial pioneers

Elisabeth Dicke and connective tissue massage

Elisabeth Dicke (1884–1952) was a physiotherapist, and following her training in the 1920s, she ran a private practice in Wuppertal Barmen. In 1929, she suffered circulatory problems and leg pain, as well as renal colic and an inflammatory swelling of the liver. She also noticed lumps in the subcutaneous tissue of the abdomen. She treated herself through self-massage, including in parts of the body that were relatively far away from the problem areas, such as the back and pelvis. According to her own reports, this enabled her to remedy the pain.

In 1938, Elisabeth Dicke and Hede Teirich-Leube developed their method of connective tissue massage. Both women were physiotherapists and assumed that the connective tissue was an organ with a connection to the somatic and autonomic nervous systems. Their assumption was supported by neurological findings of sensitive skin areas that the British neurologist Henry Head had described. The new massage technique devised by Dicke and Teirich-Leube stimulated these zones, leading to autonomic responses such as relaxation, reduced blood pressure, and a slowing of the pulse. The treatment also had an impact on the internal organs and alleviated pain.

Unfortunately, Elisabeth Dicke did not live long enough to see the success of their method: it was only after her death that connective tissue massage was medically approved and validated from a neurological and physiological perspective. In 1968, Hede Teirich-Leube received the Order of Merit for her services to medical science. She died in 1979.

In 2002, after a decade of teaching at the Rolf Institute, I treated myself to a year off in order to find answers to some of the scientific questions that had been nagging me for so long. I obtained study material from physiologists and doctors on the subject of connective tissue and attended numerous conferences. I read the works of Professor Jochen Staubesand's work from 1996 in sheer astonishment: he had shown that fascia contains cells which can contract. He believed that these were kinds of muscle cells, and he conjectured that these very cells might be controlled by the autonomic nervous system. That shocked me, and I began to call universities and look for researchers who were willing to talk to me – a mere practitioner of alternative Rolfing therapy. That was not easy. Some just laughed at me or responded neither to my phone messages nor to my string of polite letters. Finally, I met Professor Frank Lehmann-Horn at the University of Ulm, a renowned neurophysiologist who was conducting research into rare muscle diseases. He was therefore an expert in the field and regarded the muscles and fascia as one unit when it comes to body movements. He was precisely the teacher and mentor I had been looking for. He accepted my proposal to begin a program of experimental research with him, which eventually became the basis of my doctorate in human biology.

When we finally succeeded in proving in the lab at Ulm that fascial tissue reacts to certain chemical messengers and is populated by muscle-like cells that allow it to actively contract, a new path was mapped out for me. I wanted to continue working hands-on as a therapist, but I also wanted to connect with other scientific fascia researchers and gain as much insight into fascia as possible. There are a few examples I would like to mention here: findings that are crucial pieces in the big puzzle that fascia researchers are currently working on.

Revolutionary discoveries

I have been working at the University of Ulm since 2003, and now work in a private research group, the Fascia Research Project, which I run together with Dr Werner Klingler. Recent scientific fascia research has emerged from many areas of medicine – histology, physiology, anatomy and neurology. Moreover, since the development of new imaging and molecular techniques, the exploration of fascia has naturally gone much deeper than it did at the beginning of the 20th century. I will mention just a few findings and discoveries by colleagues in recent years.

▶ The deep fascia in the back is densely populated with pain receptors and is therefore a potential site of pain, as shown by the pain researcher Siegfried Mense in Heidelberg.

▶ Fascia forms an expansive network that travels through the entire body, as described by Helene Langevin from Vermont, USA. A neurophysiologist and Harvard professor of alternative therapies, Helene also conducts research into acupuncture, yoga and other methods. Moreover, she has been able to prove a correlation between the fascial crossing points and the meridians, as they are known in the Chinese therapy of acupuncture. The success of acupuncture can partly be explained by its effect on fascia and its provable neurobiological effects. Langevin has also contributed new insights into yoga and massage, which you can read more about in Chapter 4.

▶ Scar-like adhesions in fascia can be influenced and significantly improved by gentle massage, as the physiotherapist Susan Chapelle and the physiologist Geoffrey Bove have shown in animal studies. The animals concerned had surgical scars and fascia adhesions in the abdominal region. They were divided into two groups, and one group was gently massaged every day with techniques similar to Rolfing therapy. These animals were later found to have smaller adhesions than those which were not massaged.

▶ Fascia can contract independently and reacts to messengers that are associated with stress – a result from our work in the Fascia Research Project at the University of Ulm. This phenomenon is due to specific types of muscle cell, namely myofibroblasts, which are very tightly encased by fascial tissue, such as the large lumbar fascia. In the case of wounds, these cells are responsible for closing the tissue and forming scar tissue. These special organs of the connective tissue appear to act as a sort of mobile strike force. Myofibroblasts and the contraction of fascia during stress may also be one reason why musculoskeletal pain occurs when an individual is unhappy or under a lot of pressure.

▶ Biomechanics specialist and movement researcher Peter Huijing demonstrated that muscular energy, which is channelled through fascia, reaches the joints in a completely different way than was originally thought. For example, a significant portion of the tensile force of the contracting muscle fibres is not transferred to the nearby muscle tendons, but instead to adjacent muscles via the fascial sheaths surrounding the muscle fibres, which sometimes have a different joint function. There are also major differences

Ida Rolf, founder of Rolfing therapy and structural integration

Ida P. Rolf (1896–1979) studied biochemistry, and in 1920 she was one of the first women in the United States to receive a doctorate in this subject. She worked as a researcher at the Rockefeller Institute, examining infectious diseases and threats to public health. The institute became a centre for clinical studies. She carried out intensive work there on chemistry and medical mathematics, but also on alternative therapies, including chiropractic, osteopathy and homeopathy.

Trying out treatment methods on family members and friends, Ida Rolf developed her manual therapy and structural integration, which was later called Rolfing therapy. When someone experiences pain, poor posture and tension, this type of therapy considers the main cause to be in the connective tissue rather than in the muscles and bones. Ida Rolf was convinced that the connective tissue and the condition of the entire body can be influenced by manual therapy. She largely based her therapy on mechanical factors, because she knew that the connective tissue was a malleable material that was rich in collagen and therefore wanted to influence the tissue mainly through physical input, such as pressure and massage. As early as 1971, she considered the body to be a network of fascia. However, she also believed in the psychological effects of manual stimulation: after a successful course of Rolfing therapy, she expected that not only should a faulty posture be corrected, but the patient should also see a reduction in fear, low self-esteem and depressive moods.

Ida P. Rolf is now considered one of the pioneers of fascial therapy, with the Rolfing method now used all over the world. Researchers and therapists who work in this field include leading fascia experts, such as the rehabilitation and Rolfing specialists Thomas Findley and Thomas Myers, who developed the system of myofascial meridians.

from one person to another. The way fascia is connected within the bodies of individuals also plays a role. Huijing's research on the role of fascia in children with spastic paralysis has been recognised with international awards.

New findings from all corners of the world are added to this list on a daily basis. Above all, there are also many practical applications, whether on the diagnosis side of things – such as a new ultrasound machine that also shows images of soft tissue such as fascia – or on the therapy side, such as treatments for patients with lower back pain, for whom neither strength training nor pain relievers have been of much benefit. More and more orthopaedic pain clinics are now shifting towards not just examining and x-raying the intervertebral discs in patients with acute back pain, but also using ultrasound and palpation diagnostics to examine the lumbar fascia. Our Ulm research group works very closely with various pain specialists and manufacturers of medical devices. Fascia may well provide an explanation for the many cases of chronic lower back pain, which is the most common complaint within the general population.

The number of interoceptors in fascia far exceeds the number of proprioceptors and mechanoreceptors (for movement, position, pressure, etc.). This highlights the great importance of these signals for the state and activity of the organs in the body. Our 'gut feeling', as in our internal awareness of our bodily functions and organ activities, seems to depend largely on the fascia – the connective tissue around the intestines.

The signals from these nerve endings travel through the spinal cord to the brain, where they enter the insula – a small region of the cerebral cortex. Incidentally, this also happens to be the region that, according to neurologists, accounts for our sense of self and our emotional state. In this way, what we call consciousness could be dependent on our internal physical awareness – and in fact on the perception and processing of numerous signals from our fascia.

Today, mental illnesses such as depression and anxiety disorder are already viewed as disorders of interoception and, as we have seen, it is the neurophysiological signals sent by interoceptors in the fascia that are responsible for this sense of internal awareness.

The human subcutaneous connective tissue plays an interesting role here. This tissue has a special sensory system for touch that indicates affection. This means greater sensitivity to skin contact, stroking

Fascial pioneers

Andrew Taylor Still, the founder of osteopathy

Andrew Taylor Still (1828–1917) was a field physician and natural healer in the United States who had no formal training. He learned the basic medical principles from his father – who himself was a doctor – and took a few courses at various institutes. He was not a graduate of a regular course of study. At his practice, he mostly worked using naturopathic methods such as cupping, blood-letting, leeching and diets, but he was also sympathetic to esoteric influences such as phrenology, mesmerism and spiritualism.

In 1870, Andrew Taylor Still turned to manual methods and undertook anatomical studies on his own initiative. In doing so, he discovered that treatments using his hands had great benefit to his patients. In patients with certain diseases, he found hard lumps in the muscles or in the skin, which could be influenced by pressure and massage, to some extent merely laying his hands on the patient's body. This is how he developed the principles of his teachings about the healing powers of the organism, which had to be triggered by touch, as well as about the fundamental importance of exercise for the human body.

In 1892, he and his family founded a school in Kansas for the treatment that Still himself called osteopathy. As one of the very first innovators, Still emphasised that the fascial tissue is supplied by nerves and is to be regarded as a sensory organ. Some of his intuitive insights into fascia as a member of the body's entire regulation system and the autonomic nervous system have now been confirmed by physiologists.

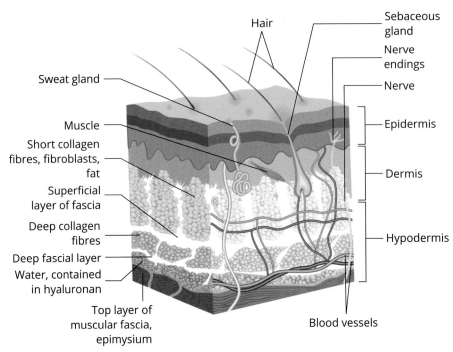

Hair

Sebaceous gland

Nerve endings

Sweat gland

Nerve

Muscle

Epidermis

Short collagen fibres, fibroblasts, fat

Superficial layer of fascia

Dermis

Deep collagen fibres

Deep fascial layer

Water, contained in hyaluronan

Hypodermis

Top layer of muscular fascia, epimysium

Blood vessels

A cross section through the skin, showing the fascial layers – superficial and deep fascia.

and body heat. This system is also connected to the brain; again to the insula, which explains why it also influences our emotional state, sense of empathy and interpersonal skills.

Have I raved on about the paramount importance of fascia enough yet? As you can probably tell, I am so fascinated by the world of fascia that I have to remind myself to come up for air every now and then. Partly responsible for this are my many dedicated and inspiring colleagues around the world, who are all sharing their findings with one another

and working together to establish a new representation of the body as the complex network we now know it to be. The pioneering spirit that characterises this field is infectious – and I can't deny that it gives me great pleasure. In the year 2000 or so when I tried to make contact with researchers and scientists in this field, I came up against many closed doors and had to wait a long, long time to get an appointment or a meeting, if at all. Today, those same researchers call on me and my colleagues in fascia research for knowledge and advice.

New perspectives on back pain – the suffering we share

Chronic back pain is something many of us now suffer from and one of the most common causes of disability and early retirement. And yet, we still have no adequate explanation as to what causes it. The usual suspects are intervertebral discs, vertebrae, nerves or weak and incorrectly exercised muscles. Only very rarely do disc and vertebral operations lead to permanent improvement. Conversely, there are many people with visible intervertebral disc and vertebral damage who have no symptoms or pain. Muscle strengthening does not always help – even well-trained athletes can suffer from back pain.

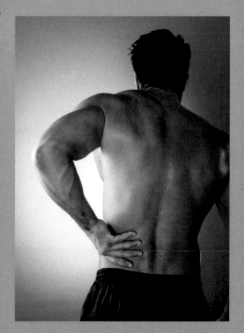

Fascia research is shedding new light on the problem. Firstly, we have learned that the fascial tissue is densely populated with pain sensors, especially in the back. We then saw that, because the large lumbar fascia contains many contractile cells, it contracts under the influence of certain substances and under stress. Studies carried out on male patients with back pain have shown that their lumbar fascia, the large fascia in the lower back region, is significantly thicker. This entire area is highly sensitive to pain, and patients tend to have a characteristic way of walking. All this suggests that disorders or problems in the fascial tissue in the back contribute to pain, or that these issues might even arise there. Small wounds or fractures in fascia caused by irregular and one-sided strain may play a key role. Such micro-injuries to the fascial tissue could cause inflammation, as well as false signals, which are then transmitted from the fascia to the muscles. The subsequent muscle disorders cause further cramping, and both of these together could lead to chronic back pain. This has given rise to researchers all over the world continuing to investigate the role of fascia in the generation of pain.

Recently, researchers in the United States have shown that lack of exercise, as well as tiny injuries to the tissue of the lumbar fascia, both play an equal part in this large fascia becoming matted. Doing less exercise may in part be due to the patient's attempts to avoid the pain, as people tend to move less when they are worried about pain. It's bad enough if the back fascia is affected by just one of these two issues – if you're something of a chronic couch potato, for example – but things get really bad when both of these factors come together. So the long and the short of it is: if you have back pain, you should definitely keep moving. Otherwise you are at risk of severe matting in the large lumbar fascia, which takes a long time to undo.

Another finding of the fascial research into back pain is that the pain deep inside the back that starts in the fascia has a very particular characteristic, in that patients often describe it as being 'nasty' or 'horrible'. People tend not to attribute these sorts of emotional attachments to muscle pain.

We also have a new understanding of how this large back fascia is structured. Researchers in the US recently found that it is made up of three different layers. The top two layers closest to the skin are actually tensed by different muscles, despite being very closely interlinked – so they slide against each other only a very minimal amount. The first of the two layers is a core component of the functional fascial line in the back, while the second is part of the large dorsal line (page 72). These findings have already impacted the exercises athletes do to prevent back problems. These days, we not only work out the back muscles themselves, but also include exercises that use the arms. The aim of this is to create an active network of tensile stress between the arms and legs and across the back, which stimulates this important layer of fascia.

The third and deepest of the three layers of fascia in the back is connected to the abdomen and thus the abdominal fascial network. This is tensed by the innermost abdominal wall muscle, which in turn is closely linked to the pelvic floor and the diaphragm. This new anatomical finding shows that exercises which stabilise the core – such as those used in Pilates – could be the ideal solution to back pain.

The exercises in this book incorporate these new findings about the deep layer of lumbar fascia and its connection to the abdomen, and you will find that some now include the pelvic floor and diaphragmatic breathing. You will learn about these in Chapter 3.

For now, I'd like to mention more about the intervertebral discs. While they often have the finger of blame pointed in their direction, they are actually only to blame for around 15 percent of back problems. And even if the source of the pain genuinely is a herniated or slipped disc, the fascia is in fact partially responsible. That is because the intervertebral discs are encased in a fibrous sheath, which is what holds them in shape. This sheath, referred to in the medical world as the *anulus fibrosus*, is a layer of tissue made up of cartilage and fascial connective tissue, and contains a high proportion of collagen. In healthy people, its fibres are arranged in a criss-crossing pattern, running diagonally to the axis of the body. Based on this, fascial experts have been able to conclude that the torso, along with its ligaments and vertebrae, is naturally configured to perform rotating movements – i.e. to rotate and twist around its own axis. One issue is that people nowadays tend not to get enough exercise, but particularly that they only perform a very limited repertoire of movements as part of their day-to-day life. This could be one reason for the degeneration of the fascial sheaths between the vertebrae. If the sheath around the vertebrae tears, the intervertebral disc pushes out. This is what is known as a herniated or slipped disc. Fascia researchers and therapists therefore believe that, in order to be effective, any training intended to prevent back pain must also include rotational movements such as barbell torso twists or oblique sit-ups. The twisting versions of the flamingo, throwing and elastic jumps exercises, which you will find in the next chapter, are ideal for this.

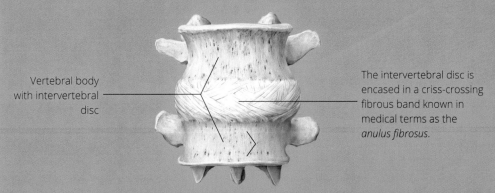

Vertebral body with intervertebral disc

The intervertebral disc is encased in a criss-crossing fibrous band known in medical terms as the *anulus fibrosus*.

The intervertebral discs between the vertebral bodies are clearly designed to account for the fact that the vertebrae are often twisted against one other, because the protective band around them is made up of criss-crossing fibres.

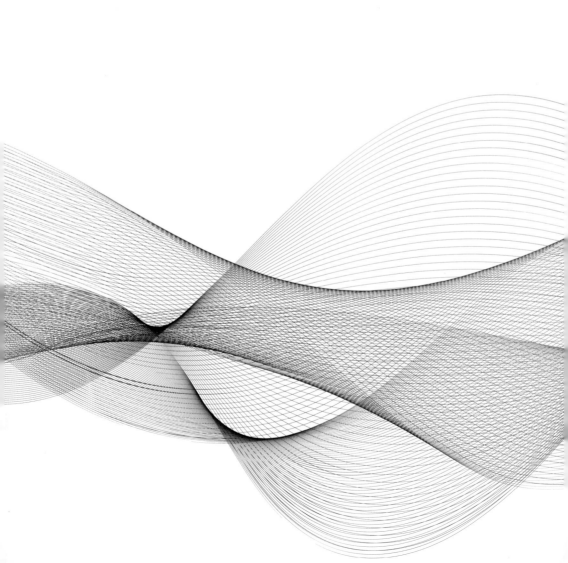

Chapter 2

The principles of
fascia training

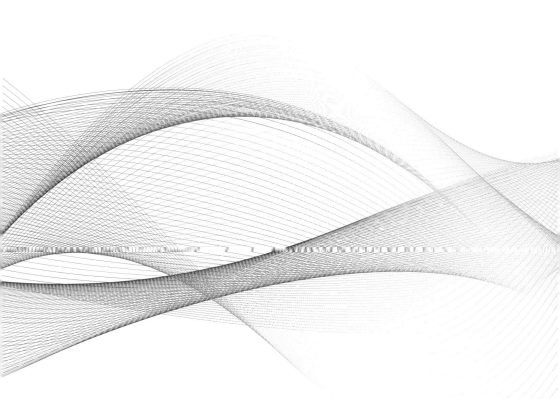

Like anything, exercise is definitely a matter of fashion. There have been many popular trends over the years such as stretching, aerobics, Callanetics, and Asian martial arts styles, as well as yoga and Pilates. There are training plans that are done with equipment or without, with a partner or alone, indoors, outdoors, with instructions, with music, with exercises to follow on screen, and with weekly schedules and diet plans. Over the course of time and as new discoveries are made, some teachings fall by the wayside while others make a resurgence. The thing to remember is that there is no set way.

And why should there be? By being open to change and adapting to the latest scientific findings, training programs can keep being improved or updated. That's exactly what has happened over the last few years, thanks to fascial research. Incorporating knowledge about the functionality of fascia can influence previous training methods and common exercise routines. That doesn't mean you have to discard or replace everything that you are used to, however, because a lot of it can be integrated into your usual routine. The new fascia exercises merely widen the spectrum – they do not radically change it. If you are clear about the role of fascia in movement, you can also improve your performance using a program that you already follow. And even if

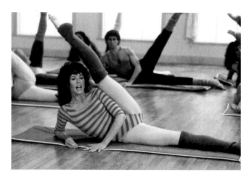

A trend from the 1980s: Jane Fonda's workout for women.

you are not currently following a training regime, you can gain a greater awareness of your fascia and learn easy exercises that will give you a brilliant introduction to healthy movement.

Fascia training does not aim to replace any previous training programs; it complements and enriches them by means of a component that has generally been missing. In other words, it simply completes the picture. Fascia training forms one element of muscular, cardiovascular and coordination training – it adds the finishing touch to your personal training program. This applies to athletes of all levels – but also to those of us who aren't athletes, too.

Healthy movement in everyday life

That is, our goal is not limited to achieving better performance in sports. The fascia workout has enormous importance for everyday movement, as well as for prevention and rehabilitation in case of injury. Healthy exercise in everyday life is particularly close to my heart. I fear that modern-day life has a very restrictive effect on our natural movement, and that we no longer move in the way that our bodies are designed for. Our capacity for movement is deteriorating, and office work requires us to sit in an unnatural, hunched position for hours on end. Staying in one position for long periods is bad for fascia, but we even cause ourselves problems when we're walking or running, too – by wearing unsuitable shoes.

Musculoskeletal pain is so widespread that it has been said that "If you're over 40 and you don't wake up in pain in the morning, you're probably dead". As we already know, changes and injuries in fascia are the likely cause of many of these pain disorders and illnesses – and that is precisely the reason why the fascial system in our body should always be well maintained. This applies particularly to people who have to spend a lot of time sitting down, because fascia needs exercise.

Especially in middle age, it becomes increasingly important to keep on top of our fascial fitness. The contorted body shape – the typical profile of an elderly person with hunched torso and forward-rounded shoulders – is to a large extent a result of ageing of fascia. The dreaded stiffness that comes with age arises from the fact that the connective tissue becomes matted with advancing years, usually due to the lack of exercise. This is not merely a cosmetic problem. Falls and injuries, as well as pain in the musculoskeletal system, are also connected with reduced mobility. If fascia is fit and in good condition, it is possible to retain a youthful, toned body shape and suppleness well into old age. So if you want to stay young, or to feel young again, you will do well to strengthen the network that is so crucial to our vitality.

You are probably familiar with the phrase 'use it or lose it!'. Well, the same principle applies to our bodies. Our bones, muscles, tendons, fascia and even our nerves

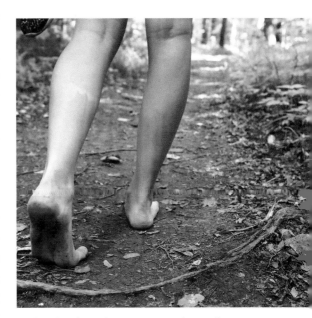

Walking barefoot is how we were made to walk. It's natural and does wonders for the fascia in your feet.

can be either built up or broken down, depending on how we use them. What we do not need or ordinarily require, the body regards as unwanted baggage and therefore tries to reduce it in order to save energy. Conversely, the muscles we do need and train on a regular basis remain intact. To combat this in old age, we can do specific exercises that affect both the number of neurons in our brain and the connections between them, in order to increase bone and muscle mass. This also applies to fascia.

What you need to know before you train

In this chapter, we will take a closer look at the function of fascia, specifically within the human musculoskeletal system. We will gain further understanding of the role it plays in muscle function, and how the muscles and fascia interact with one another. We also consider the importance of fascial tissue not only for mobility and the joints, but also for the shape of our bodies. I will be presenting you with a new representation of the body that is not based on rigid, mechanically connected bones, but rather consists of a dynamic network of long fascial lines. At the end of this chapter there is a test which you can use to determine your natural type of connective tissue. All this is important for

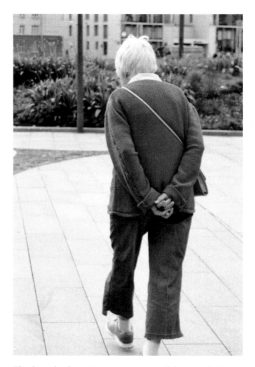

The hunched posture common in older people is due to the condition of the fascia.

selecting the exercises that you will get to know later and will hopefully try out.

If they so wish, impatient readers can – in theory – skip ahead and go directly to the exercises, which are presented in Chapter 3, along with pictures and descriptions. But to be honest, I would advise against it. It would be far better to read the following sections on the importance of fascia for human movement and then have a go at the test. What you learn here will help you to understand the exercises, and – above all – give you the motivation you need to do them!

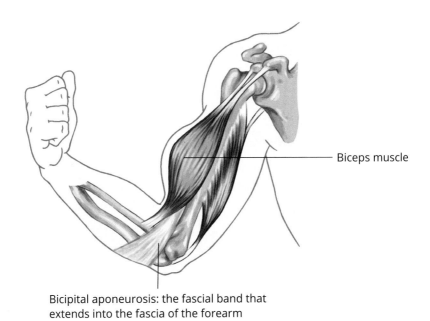

Biceps muscle

Bicipital aponeurosis: the fascial band that
extends into the fascia of the forearm

*The biceps muscle is attached to the bones of the shoulder and forearm by tendons, which give tension to the
bone. A band of fascia keeps the muscle in place below the elbow.*

How the muscles and fascia work together

As we saw in Chapter 1, muscle and fascia form a single unit. However, fascia also has distinct functions relating to movement, to structure and posture of the body, and also to body shape. We will begin with the function of fascia in the muscles themselves, where – from a purely anatomical standpoint – it exists in the form of sheaths that are encased around muscle fibres, bundles of fibre, as well as around the entire muscle. But what exactly does fascia do here?

We learned in Chapter 1 that each individual fibre of a muscle is sheathed in fascial tissue. The role that these sheaths play in energy transfer is connected to the mechanics of the muscle and the movement as a whole. In order to move the limbs, the muscles need to be connected to the bones. This connection is provided by the tendons or the plates of connective tissue called aponeuroses, whose solid fibres are fused with the periosteum or specific attachment points on the bones. They consist of tight fascial tissue containing very strong and densely packed collagen fibres.

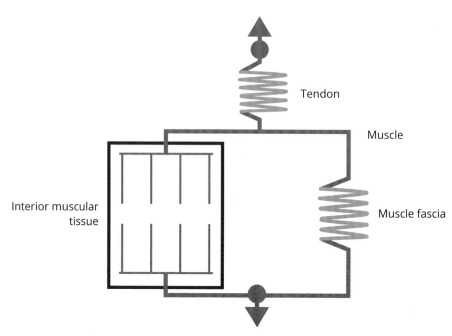

Schematic diagram of the muscle according to Hill, showing how the muscles and fascia work together. With their springy elastic properties, the blue fascial elements complement the tensile force of the muscle fibres.

There is a smooth transition between the bones and the tendon tissue: the bone attaches to the tendon via the cartilage. The tendon then attaches to the muscle, again via specialised tissue cells in the intersection between tendon and muscle. And so we have this continuum of fascial tissue, which stores and transfers the mechanical energy of the muscle.

The very fact that the force of the muscle reaches the tendon, and that this tension passes to the bone, occurs only thanks to the performance of the fascial sheaths in and around the muscle. The role that they play is to carry energy from one point to another. Fascia obtains energy from the contraction of many muscle cells and passes it on from one sheath to the next – i.e. from the endomysium to the epimysium – and then to the tendon, where the force finally reaches the bone. The effect of muscle strength is thus based specifically on the cooperation of muscle and fascia. Biomechanical engineers illustrate this using the image of a feather.

Elasticity – an integral property of fascia

Elastic springiness is a very important factor and plays a central role in fascia's ability to move. Yet the ability of a structure to spring at all means that something within it has to be elastic. In other words, the material has to be able to change its shape when a tensile force is applied, and then to return to its own shape once the tension subsides. We already know from Chapter 1 that fascial tissue is made of elastic material, primarily collagen. It is a characteristic of elastic material that the energy applied to it – in this case, the tensile force – is stored as energy and then released again. From a physical perspective, the atoms move closer together when the tensile force is applied, and return to their original positions when the force subsides. The more force that is applied to the atoms, the faster they return to their previous position, as they remain tense until they are able to release the energy that they have absorbed through the tensile force. There is a correlation between the force of the impact and the force of the rebound, which is also partially determined by the material. Elastic material with a high capacity to store energy bounces back sharply, as in the case of a metal spring. The same applies to the fascia that encases the muscles, but the tendons in particular.

Moreover, the tissue that makes up the muscle fascia is not straight like a plank of wood. Instead, the bundles of collagen fibres that comprise the muscle fascia are slightly wavy. As a result, the fascial sheath does not lie entirely flush against the muscle. The waves provide the give

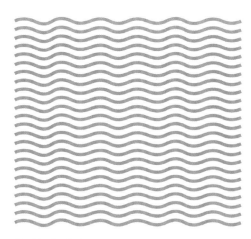

Healthy fascia has a wavy structure.

needed for the tissue to expand, as well as providing the ability to store energy. The structure has the appearance of wavy hair: the more pronounced the waves are, the more springy and elastic the fascia will be.

With age, this wavy structure significantly decreases, as in turn does the elasticity of the fascia. However, it is possible to delay this process. A British study that I found particularly fascinating was able to demonstrate that, with the right training, the wavy shape of the fascial tissue can be restored after only a few months – even in older subjects. In other words, exercises that effectively train the elastic storage capacity of fascia not only make our movements more springy, but also restore springiness in the architecture of our fascial tissue.

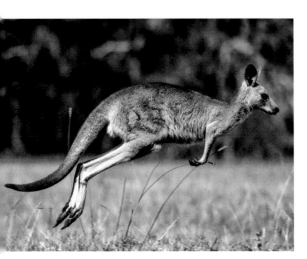 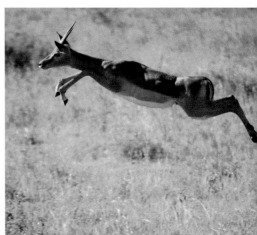

When they jump, kangaroos use the tendons in their long hind legs to bounce off the ground. Gazelles are the masters of the high jump and the long jump.

Springiness and the ability to develop elastic force and recharge with energy are essential features of the fascia and tendons. Both of these properties allow for elastic movements and outstanding performance, as biomechanical engineers have found from observing antelopes and kangaroos. These animals are able to jump incredibly high and far. Small antelopes manage to jump to a height of 3 m and a distance of 10 m, while red kangaroos can jump distances of more than 13 m, which is further than any other animal. The red kangaroo can also run as fast as a racehorse – up to 60 km per hour.

This extraordinary performance, however, cannot be explained solely by muscle strength. Antelopes and gazelles, for example, are delicate creatures and do not have large muscle masses, but their graceful limbs do have long tendons. Kangaroos have remarkably long hind legs and very strong Achilles tendons. In fact, it is this combination of the strong tendons and the long legs of both kangaroos and antelopes that is responsible for their amazing performance. The huge leaps that these animals can make are due to the ingenious mechanism of fascia.

The catapult effect

How the spring effect works can be explained biomechanically by comparing it to the mechanism of a catapult. A catapult hurls an object forward as a result of the mechanical tension applied to it. When this tension is suddenly discharged, the stored energy is transformed into kinetic energy, and the load is propelled forward. Another very simple example is a rubber band which is stretched and then quickly released. Or a rubber ball: when a rubber ball drops to the ground, the impact exerts pressure onto the ball, which then deforms and charges up with tensile energy. It then snaps back to its original shape and springs back up from the ground.

This catapult effect therefore makes it possible to move around with a minimum degree of muscle strength. The muscles also produce a triggering contraction, which puts tension on the tendons. After

Catapults, which were used as long-range weapons in the Middle Ages, produce a high degree of tensile energy.

the initial jump, all the subsequent jumps rely mainly on gravity and the weight of the body. When the body bounces back onto the floor, the ankle and the Achilles tendon compress and reload with energy. The combined energy then discharges, and the rebound may have an acceleration that exceeds the rate of speed of highly trained muscles. Animals such as gazelles, antelopes and kangaroos jump in a very energy-efficient way, mainly because their muscles are not functioning at full strength. Instead, their tendons are repeatedly absorbing and releasing mechanical force.

The mechanism is slightly different when something jumps from a standing position, such as a frog leaping suddenly into the air, or a cat jumping from the ground onto a high wall. In this instance, the animal pre-loads its muscles by crouching down and briefly tensing all the muscles connected to its long tendons. In preparation for the jump, the muscles twitch as quickly as possible, the tendons bounce back even more quickly – and the animal takes off.

This catapult effect of the tendons and fascia is a universal biomechanical principle in animals – and in humans too. When we humans hop and jump, as well as when we walk or run, we too benefit from this catapult effect. Biomechanical engineers

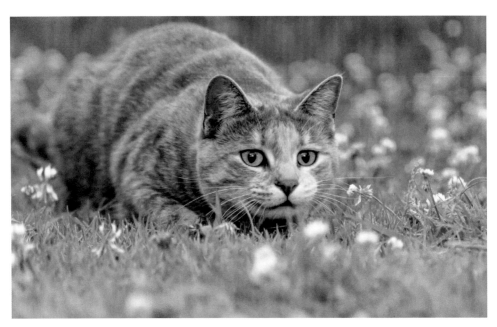

Ready to pounce: the cat crouches, tenses its muscles and loads its tendons with tensile energy.

have discovered that the ability of fascia to store mechanical energy is very similar between humans and gazelles. The capacity of our tendons to store energy even surpasses that of all other primates. Humans are the only primates that have those gazelle-like tendons in their legs that make us so good at running and jumping. This shows that Homo sapiens have evolved to a much greater degree than their climbing relatives.

Walking: a very human specialism

Humans are known to show particular endurance when it comes to walking. We can go for hours with almost no fatigue. This is hardly surprising, since – as researchers have discovered – the muscles have far less work to do in bipeds walking upright than in our primate relatives, who walk using all four limbs, placing their knuckles on the ground as they go. This is mainly due to the springy catapult mechanism from which we benefit. The same applies to jogging, with people generally being able to keep up a relatively fast-paced jog for fairly long periods.

This miracle of movement happens because of a chain of fascia, which spans from the large plantar fascia in our feet to the Achilles tendon on the heel, via a musculofascial chain all the way up to our back. Fascia and muscles work together in units, with two points of attachment on each bone.

Since this chain of fascial tissue can store a lot of energy and subsequently release it without any muscular intervention, the human gait is very efficient and enduring. We will talk more about gait, feet, walking and running later in this chapter, and you can also find out more about this in Chapter 4, as fascia research has shed new light on these areas, too.

So, we now that we need to exercise our fascia and keep it fit in order to maintain and improve its elasticity and energy storage capacity. Only those tendons and fascia that are in good shape and have the right structure can efficiently store energy and release it again.

Fascial lines and the tension network

The wide-ranging mechanics of fascia, as I have described with reference to walking and the lumbar fascial line, influence the types of exercise that we deem necessary. As we have seen, walking involves far more of our fascia than just the fascia in our feet – and this principle applies to the fascia in the body as a whole. There are long chains of musculofascial units that run through the body like railway lines, and are responsible for posture, stability and efficient, fluid motion.

It is only fairly recently that these long musculofascial chains have been discovered and identified as an important part of training. A particularly plausible and detailed model for this system was developed by my Rolfing colleague Thomas W. Myers, who has been working on it since the 1990s. Myers is a Rolfing therapist and we taught anatomy together at the Ida Rolf Institute. He also trained with the architect Richard Buckminster-Fuller and physicist Moshé Feldenkrais, and has a deep understanding of many of the procedures used in physiotherapy. His system of long musculofascial chains in the body, which was derived purely from practical work, has now been acknowledged in its many

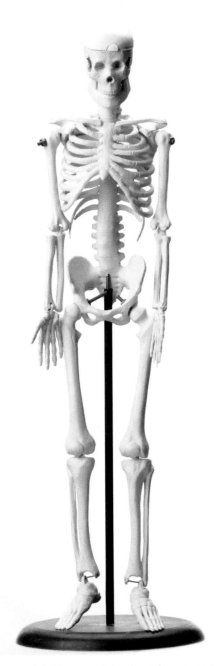

A skeleton cannot stand upright on its own – it always needs a prop, as this model shows.

aspects, and has also been extensively confirmed by medics and anatomists.

The skeleton is not what holds us up

Myers' model is based on the notion that it is not the bones that keep the body upright and supported, but primarily the fascia. This is evidenced by the fact that a skeleton cannot stand erect unaided; without support it would simply fall apart. The skeleton is not designed like scaffolding – a stable structure that provides support to adjacent parts.

The main thing that keeps the body upright is in fact the fascia and muscles together that make up a dynamic network of tension. We know, for instance, that remaining upright requires small but constant adjustments in muscle tension and automatic balancing. If we didn't do this, we would simply fall to the ground. We can't stand up when we're asleep due to the lack of muscular tension. The muscle tension, in turn, is transferred through the fascia, which also provides additional independent elements within this network.

The sailboat principle: the spine

Info

For several years, medical and orthopaedic practitioners have used the image of a sailboat with its mast, shrouds and rigging to describe the static conditions in the spine. The role of the mast is to provide a stable element within a system of tension. The stability is provided by the ropes pulling in various directions to moor the mast in place. A similar principle applies to our backs. In the back, there are ligaments and muscles which are tensed, keeping the spine upright. In the middle runs the deep back extensor. This draws the movable – and wobbly – segments of vertebrae together and stabilises them. There are then additional elements that pull out to the sides, reinforcing the back's dynamic load-bearing capacity.

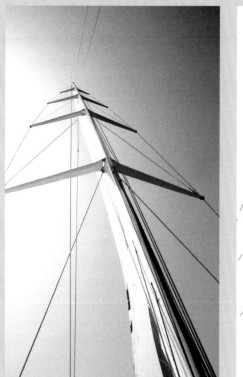 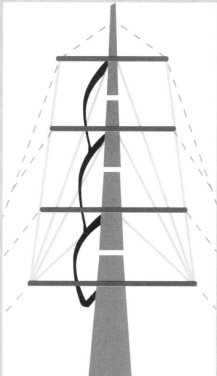

The mast of a sailing yacht represents the spine (left). The tension system of the spine, from a medical perspective (right).

The tensegrity model

These types of tension networks also exist within architecture, in the design of static structures. Here they are known as 'tensegrity models', 'tensegrity' being a made-up term derived from the words 'tension' and 'integrity'. These structures were first developed in the mid-20th century by American artists and architects, and have the following characteristics:

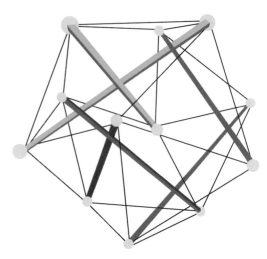

The tensegrity model. It is the tension that makes these systems both stable and dynamic.

- ▶ The structure consists of stable and elastic elements.
- ▶ The elastic elements are in a state of tension.
- ▶ The stable elements are connected to one another only by elastic elements.
- ▶ The stable elements do not have direct connections to anywhere.
- ▶ The elastic elements provide tension throughout the system.

Fascia researchers believe that the key aspects of human body structure conform with the tensegrity principle, with long musculofascial chains forming a tension network with the bones. This system is highly responsive to movement; it is dynamic. If we activate a muscle in one place, a reaction somewhere else in the body is triggered through the long fascia chain to which it is connected. Muscles do not work independently; they are always linked together in the body's fascial network. This way of thinking goes beyond the classical anatomical theory of individually localised muscles, and identifies larger functional fascial units in the body.

A new way of looking at the body

This new way of looking at the human body has important implications, such as for our understanding of the bones and joints. We now understand, for example, that there are very few places in the body where the bones actually touch one another directly. In actual fact, they are connected with connective tissue – cartilage, capsules, ligaments and tendons, allowing for flexible movement. When you start looking at the body this way, you automatically see the spinal column differently, too. As described earlier in the chapter, the spine is not a central pillar like in an ancient temple, but rather just one of the stable elements in a larger support structure – albeit a very special one, due to its extreme flexibility. Our spinal column is not a column at all, but more like a flexible chain. That is because the backbone is not actually one continuous bone, like the femur, but instead comprises several individual elements, all held together by ligaments and a whole system of fascia and small muscles. We therefore prefer the term 'spinal chain' rather than spinal column.

Fascia researchers now view all issues of body posture and upright walking in terms of the dynamic network that runs throughout the body, especially in the back. In our research group in Ulm, Germany, we are particularly interested in developing new models of human gait based on this new understanding, as well as with the causes of deep lower back pain, which may also be due to the dynamics of the fascial network.

Fascial lines and their route through the body

As we have seen, our body is made up of a whole network of different tensile elements, within which some larger, long musculofascial chains can now be identified. We believe that these myofascial meridians play a special role in our coordination and the suppleness of our movements. They therefore need to be triggered and activated during exercise, so that we can achieve good coordination and proper function throughout the entire chain. Isolated exercises for individual muscle groups, as are used in typical strength training, are not adequate. From the perspective of fascial research, the remote connections between muscle and tissue around the body are just as important. We want to be focusing on these as part of our training, and so we will now give you a brief overview of the eight most important fascial lines in the body.

Fascia research has now produced some pretty reliable evidence in relation to these lines. A lot has changed since this book was first published in 2014, with research having enriched the field significantly in the intervening years. For example, in 2014, we had still only recorded six of these lines. We have now expanded this to include eight major lines, including two spanning the back, one across the abdominal area and arms, and one that runs diagonally across the torso. These trajectories each run over several body parts and extremities, and play a role in providing both support and movement. While their functions have been defined in great detail by Thomas Myers – with Jan Wilke also building on this work – for the purpose of this book, we will be looking at just the most important keywords. If you want to dig deeper into the topic, you will find suggestions for further reading in the appendix.

1. Large dorsal line

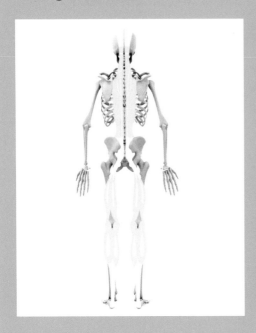

The large dorsal line runs from the thick fascia on the sole of the foot known as the plantar fascia, through the heel pads, Achilles tendon and calves, then over the back and neck and up to the skull. It supports the back and is responsible for maintaining an upright posture.

2. Functional dorsal line

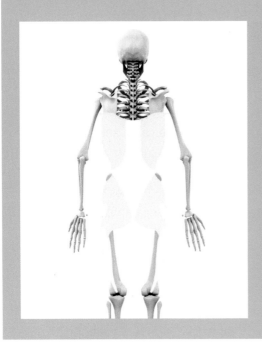

A second chain runs up the back of the body, covering the torso, buttocks and thighs. It connects the upper body with the lower body in movements involving the arms and legs. It also helps to stabilise the back.

3. Arm–chest–abdomen line

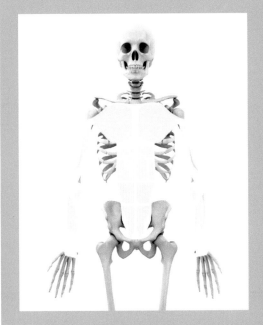

This front line connects the chest, stomach and arms on the front of the body, down to the sternum. It combines two lines previously depicted by Thomas Myers, namely the 'superficial front arm line' (SFAL) and the 'front functional line' (FFL). This plays a significant role in movements involved in climbing, hanging and similar.

4. Diagonal torso line

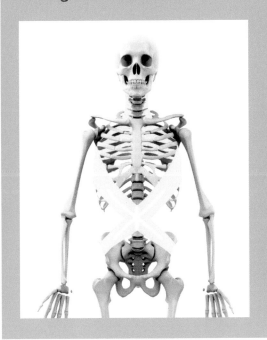

This line winds like a spiral around the entire torso. When walking, it ensures dynamic rotation between the pelvis and the rib cage. It also plays an important role in the throwing action – when you lunge one arm forward, while playing rounders, for example. Another example of this can be seen when a footballer takes a power shot, where there is usually a pronounced swivel of the torso in the direction of the goal.

5. Shoulder–elbow line

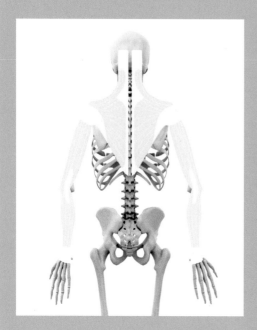

This line runs from the outer side of the forearm and upper arm, up to the deltoid muscle, which encases the entire shoulder joint. There, it passes into the fascia of the trapezius muscle, which connects the line to the back of the head, covering a large proportion of the back in between.

6. Adductors–pelvic floor line

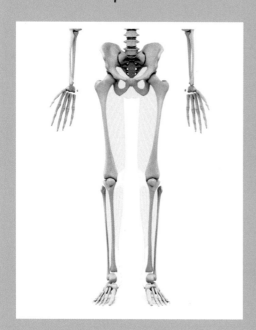

This line is shared by humans and some marsupials. It connects the insides of the legs with the front of the pelvic floor. It also stabilises the knee joints and ensures good pelvic stability in sports and day-to-day activities.

7. Abdominal net

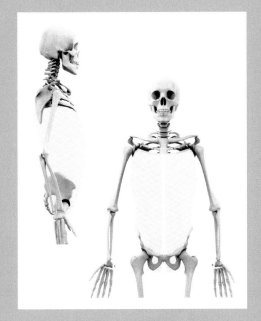

This line is like a girdle of fascia, that extends from the middle of the abdomen to the large back fascia known as the *thoracolumbar fascia*. It is made up of several layers of fascial tissue, which surround and interlink the straight, oblique and transverse abdominal muscles. Like a corset, it tightens and draws together the tummy, chest and back. This fascial abdominal tension plays an important role in the stability of the back.

8. Lateral line

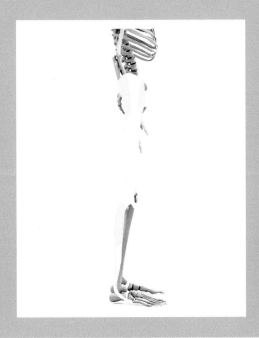

The lateral lines encase the outsides of the hips and legs. On the foot, they pull from the outside of the foot, around the ankle to the sole, where they are connected to the thick plantar fascia. The two lateral lines play a major role in many of the movements involving the legs and pelvis, as well as for balancing on one leg.

Fascial lines in motion

In certain movements, the long fascial lines are even visible; they can be observed, for example, in javelin or discus throwing, in swinging movements and in certain forms of gymnastics. These types of movement were formerly part of the exercise repertoire, as historical images show, but today these poses look somewhat out of date.

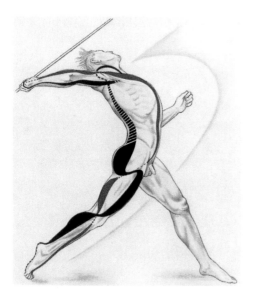
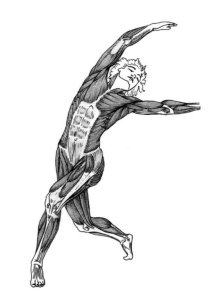

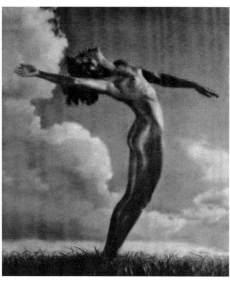
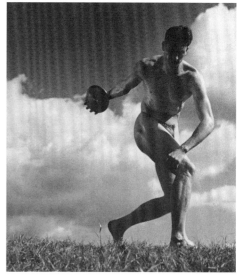

Anatomical illustrations of fascial lines compared with sports and gymnastics poses.

Old-school gymnastics

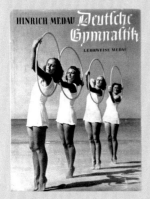

Our grandparents and great-grandparents will have been very familiar with the aerobic exercises that we now know focus on the long fascial lines, especially those which involve swinging, rhythmic movements that stimulate the entire body. This form of physical education became accessible to both men and women in the 19th century with the advent of modern gymnastics, and was especially popular during the first half of the century. Exercises involved swinging or throwing balls, tyres and bats, whereby participants stretched and bent themselves energetically in all directions.

The title of Hinrich Medau's book from 1940.

These forms of gymnastics have a long tradition and include elements borrowed from dance, remedial exercises and coordination sports like fencing. The dancer Rudolf von Laban (1879–1958) was a co-founder of one of the schools that taught these disciplines. Hinrich and Senta Medau, who were music and gym teachers, founded their own school in the 1920s to teach holistic movement classes involving dance, full-body stretching and swinging.

Despite seeming quite old-fashioned now, these exercises clearly trigger the long fascial lines and the ligament system, especially in the back – although, back then, the teachers of the discipline were not necessarily aware of this. In the course of modern sports science, the popularity of these sorts of exercises fizzled out in the 1970s. It was widely believed that they exert excessive shearing forces on the joints and especially on the spinal column, which is at best ineffective and at worst could lead to injuries. This old style of gymnastics that involved lots of swinging has since been replaced with exercises that systematically activate either the individual muscles or the cardiovascular system. However, fascia researchers believe that this is not the right way. They want to bring back elements of bouncing and swinging, which is why we recommend it as part of the exercises in this book. Incidentally, few people know that these older European gymnastic movements actually had an influence on Indian yoga positions. That's because, during the colonial era, Europeans brought their exercise regimes over to India, where they continued to be developed. There will be more on this in Chapter 4.

Some of our fascia exercises are similar to the swinging exercises used in traditional gymnastics. Older sport doctrines and exercise regimes made significant use of the long fascial lines, but these have been somewhat forgotten within modern sports science.

How does connective tissue respond to training?

Fascia is alive, and as such it responds to stimuli and adapts to stresses. Therefore, targeted and regular training of fascia works, because it slowly but sustainably changes the tissue. Animal studies have shown that this improves the elastic properties of the tissue and its ability to bounce back. Rats that were made to run on a wheel regularly had tighter fascia, which would spring back into shape better when pulled than the tissue of rats that were not made to run.

If it sits, it sticks!!

Fascial tissue degenerates if it is not exercised. Remember the "use it or lose it" concept mentioned earlier? Well, this also applies to the fascia. These microscopic images taken by Japanese researchers show what happens when our bodies are inactive for a long period: fascia becomes really matted.

When the fascia matt up and stick together in this way, it restricts our muscle function because the bundles of fibre are no longer able to slide past each other properly. This also interferes with the smooth transfer of energy from one muscle to the next, which in turn affects our coordination. This reduces the fluidity of our movements and uses up more energy. Our posture takes a hit too, as the reduced elasticity of the matted tissue makes us stiff. We now know that the majority of patients who suffer from back pain also have thickening and matting of the lumbar fascia. Matted fascial tissue is also a sign of ageing. Young people tend to have an even, regular tissue structure, while the fascia of the elderly (who are less active) tends to be tangled and matted together, thus losing its wavy structure.

Some of these phenomena are natural because the connective tissue cells produce more collagen when ageing. However, the replacement and decomposition of old fibres occurs more slowly, the tissue does not get renewed as dynamically as before, and there is less water in the matrix. Exercise is very effective at delaying or even reversing these symptoms, as it encourages the cells to produce new collagen, and the decomposition of old collagen is accelerated. We are already aware of such effects from muscular research: as we age, the muscles naturally waste away, but through exercise this process can be

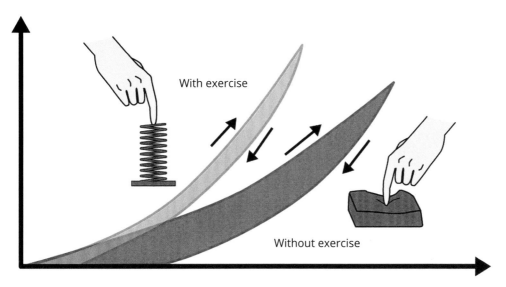

In the animals that have been exercised (blue), the tissue yields less easily under pressure – it springs back. The tissue of the animals that have not been exercised – image and curve on the right, grey – is easy to push in and is inert, in that it takes a long time to return to its shape and does not spring back. In addition, the fascia of the exercised animals has a higher maximum energy storage capacity.

halted. Even among elderly people, lost muscle mass can be rebuilt. By the same measure, we can also continue to train our fascia well into old age, keeping it firm, healthy and elastic. The more we mobilise and train our fascia – in the right way, of course – the longer it will work for us.

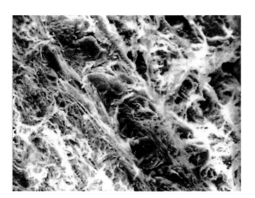
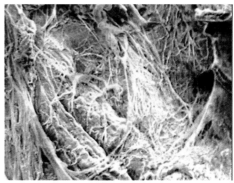

The image on the left shows normal fascial tissue in the lower leg; on the right, you can see the fascia in a leg that has been in a cast for several weeks.

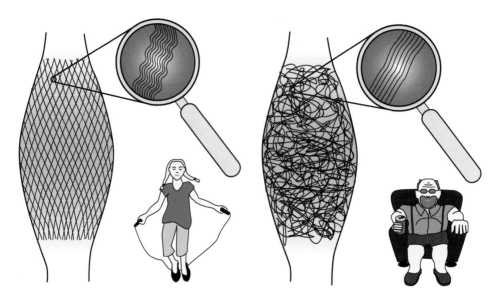

In older people, the fascia becomes matted not only as a sign of old age (right), but also as a result of reduced mobility. In addition, the fibre bundles lose the youthful waviness that allows for supple, springy movements.

Fascia training takes time

Fascia does respond to training, but not in the same way as muscle. The conversion rate of fascia is not as high as that of muscle, in that connective tissue fibres take longer to renew than muscles take to grow. However, when the connective tissue cells receive the right stimuli, their metabolism is boosted and they produce new fibres, which then reconnect and rearrange themselves in the wave-like structure that is typical of healthy tissue. The structure of fascia changes its length, strength and lubricity to adapt to the daily stresses and strains to which it is subjected. If tensile force is frequently applied, the connective tissue cells linking the bands within the tissue become tighter or are even completely replaced. This results in significantly higher elastic storage capacity – in other words, a greater capacity to act as a spring. Even if the tissue has been neglected for some time, perhaps because a limb has been in a plaster cast, proper training can reactivate the matted tissue.

You only need to look at an athlete to see how well fascia can adapt to stress. Runners and tennis players, who put immense strain on their muscles and joints, especially when stopping, have firm, tight lateral thigh fascia, for example. This fascia, known as the fascia lata, is particularly pronounced on the outside of the thigh, giving the outer thigh a much flatter appearance when seen from the front. Even in non-athletes, the normal strain of walking has a similar effect, which we know by studying the thigh fascia of wheelchair users. Their fascia is much thinner to that of people who are able to walk but do not partake in sports. The situation is different in horse riding, however, because riders use the muscles on the inside of the thigh – the adductors. As a result, fascia here becomes very strong. This affects the shape of the thigh, with horse riders' thighs often having a significant inward curve at the part of the thigh where the adductors meet the pubic bone.

Sports injuries involving fascia

For those who want to avoid injuries – particularly athletes – the condition of the fascial network is vitally important. When you see a footballer hobbling to the edge of the pitch in pain or even having to be taken off; when tennis players have to retire due to shoulder pain, or when runners pull out shortly after the start of a race, the fascial tissue is usually the culprit. Whether it is the ligaments, tendons, muscle fascia or joints, they are all susceptible to sprains, tears or capsule injuries. In most cases, injuries occur as a result of the body being subjected to a level of strain that it is not strong enough to tolerate, or because the particular region has suffered an injury in the past.

These sorts of strain injuries occur mainly to the white tissue, i.e. the fascia, and less often to the red muscle tissue. Specific fascia training can therefore protect athletes against injury, because healthy fascia is more resilient, more elastic, more stable and regenerates much faster.

Good news for sore muscles

With regard to regeneration after training and exercise, fascia research has shed new light on a phenomenon that has so far baffled us, despite being such a common complaint – and that is muscle ache.

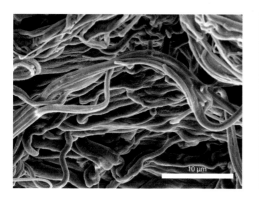 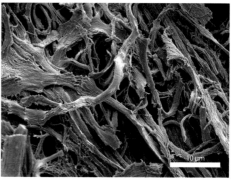

Young and old: comparison of the fibres of a six-year-old subject (left) and a 90-year-old subject (right).

Fascia matters in top athletes

I am sometimes drafted in to advise on issues relating to the fascia of top athletes. In the spring of 2015, for example, I received a call from Martin Fischer, an evolutionary biologist from the University of Jena, Germany. He had been asked to advise a javelin thrower who wanted to participate in the 2016 Olympics. The matter in question was the fascia in his throwing arm and shoulder, which the athlete, Thomas Röhler, wanted to train in a more targeted way. I then had the pleasure of being part of the team of experts supporting him during his preparation for the Olympics. Thomas Röhler had already been focusing a lot on achieving maximum rebound of the fascial elements in his throwing arm. First, I examined the fascia involved in the throwing mechanism using a portable ultrasound device. I was absolutely thrilled with the results – never before had I seen such strong and healthy-looking fascia with such clear edges on a person's upper body. That was also interesting for Thomas Röhler and his coaching team, not least because it confirmed that he was already training this fascia very effectively. In addition, it motivated us to work on developing training methods that would allow Röhler to increase the elasticity of his fascia even more over the next few years. Incidentally, Röhler won the gold medal for javelin at the 2016 Olympic Games – with a remarkable throwing distance of 90.30 metres.

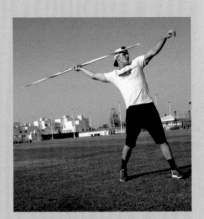

Thomas Röhler – Gold medallist at the 2016 Olympics in Rio de Janeiro.

This regularly occurs following overexertion or activities the body is not used to – particularly after braking movements, such as when walking downhill. Various explanations have been put forward over the years, be it too much lactic acid that deposits crystals that irritate the muscles, inflammation caused by free radicals, metabolic factors, cramps or tears in the muscle fibres. However, none of these theories have ever been able to adequately explain the phenomenon of muscle ache. The lactic acid theory prevailed for a long time, but has since been disproved since it became clear that muscle ache also occurs even when only minor levels of lactate are produced. In addition, the amount of lactate in the body is reduced by half after about

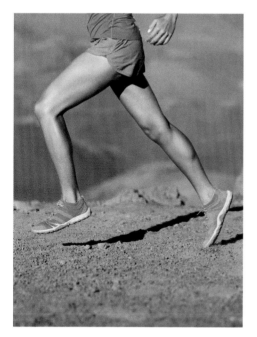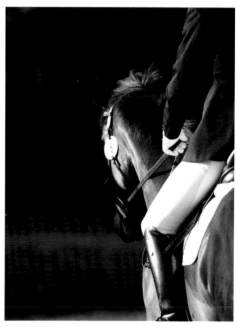

Runners and tennis players have very firm fascia in their outer thighs. Horse riders close their legs around the horse, which strengthens the fascia on the inner thigh.

20 minutes, whereas muscle ache can be delayed by one or two days, and can last for several days after that.

However, the theory that muscle ache is caused by tears in the muscles is still prevalent in conventional teachings of sports science. Among other things, this leads to the belief that it is not beneficial to massage sore muscles, as the tears are in fact injuries that would be exacerbated by massaging them. It is thought that these tears occur in the muscle fibres, followed by mild oedema and inflammation. This theory originated from a classic laboratory experiment, which showed that little tears appear in the muscle fibres when they are subjected to excessive strain. However, the level of stress applied to the muscles during these experiments far exceeds the strain that they are usually subjected to in sports. For serious researchers, it therefore remained open whether these micro-tears also appear during the level of exertion that occurs in normal exercise, when doing manual work or when walking downhill.

The part of the muscle where the soreness originates initially appeared to be a certain proportion of the muscle fibrils – specifically, the structural proteins in the red tissue, which we came across in Chapter 1: actin and titin. But that's not all, as the

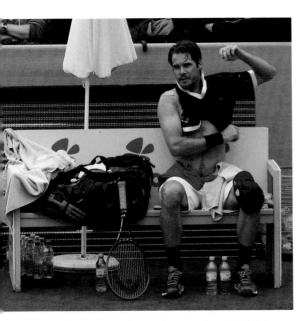

Tennis player Tommy Haas was forced to leave the court at the French Open in spring 2014 because of overstretched tendons in his shoulder. In professional tennis, impact forces can reach speeds of up to 230 km/h, which the fascial tissue of the shoulder capsule has to absorb.

order to pinpoint the origin of the pain. Investigations using saline solution in this way are an accepted procedure in pain research. In wounds and inflammation, the saline solution increases the intensity at the site of the pain, and therefore indicates where it originates from and what causes it.

Following our discussion about the role of fascia, Thomas Graven-Nielsen, a Danish pain researcher, did not hesitate in adjusting the set-up of the experiment. He and his colleague William Gibson, an Australian physiotherapy specialist, kept the main set-up of the experiment, in which test subjects were asked to climb up and down on one side of a stool for a long duration in order to induce muscle soreness in the subjects' thighs. However, only some of the subjects with muscle soreness then had saline solution injected deep into their muscular tissue. In a change to the original plan, the rest of the subjects had saline solution injected into the fascial tissue just above the thigh muscle. The results were clear: the subjects who had saline solution injected into the fascia, rather than the muscle, felt significantly more pain under pressure and movement, i.e. more muscle soreness. Admittedly, the test subjects were unable to differentiate whether their pain was coming from the muscle itself or the fascia – they simply felt that "their muscle hurt". The researchers, on the other hand, could see a clear difference. They had

fascial tissue outside the muscle plays an even bigger role. New studies have shown that the fascial sheaths around the muscles – the epimysia – are evidently the main source of the sensation of pain in sore muscles.

The early history of this discovery can be traced back to a conference in 2007, when I was joined on the panel by a selection of pain and muscle researchers. We discussed the study they had planned, which aimed to explore the cause of muscle soreness. The plan was to inject saline solution into the muscles of subjects suffering from muscle ache in injected the pain-enhancing saline solution into different locations in order to distinguish between the muscle and the fascia, and finally the mystery was solved.

This result caused quite a sensation in 2009, and since then the notion of the fascial tissue being the origin of muscle soreness has been gradually gaining more recognition. We now know that changes and injuries to the fascial tissue are the predominant cause of muscle ache. The irritation that we feel as muscle soreness arises primarily from the sheath around the muscle and not from the muscle itself. It is still unclear whether muscle ache occurs because of the suspected tears, oedema or inflammation in the fascia rather than in the muscle, or whether the pain is only perceived in the fascia because that is where all the pain sensors are. However, we do know that the feeling of muscle soreness is significantly stronger in the fascial sheath – the epimysium – than in the red muscle tissue itself.

Anyone who has ever experienced muscle soreness knows that the pain tends to go away on its own after a few days, which is how long it takes for fascia to recover. It is clear that fascia adapts to any new strain to which it is subjected, which also protects against new muscle soreness. You can find out more about this in the training principles below, as well as in the exercises in Chapter 3. For now, we can say that the new-found knowledge we have

Goals of fascia training

The things we want to achieve through our training are:

▶ optimum energy storage capacity
▶ elasticity and tensile strength
▶ smooth functioning of the long fascial lines
▶ a youthful network and wave-like structure of fascia, and
▶ speedy regeneration of the musculofascial unit following exertion.

about the role of fascia in muscle soreness has changed both the theory and the methods of treating sore muscles, which also has implications for its prevention. Healthy, fit fascia is less prone to muscle ache, which is another good reason for targeted fascia training.

Everything you need to know about fascia training

Fascia training is not the same as muscle training. Many muscle exercises in conventional programs move and exercise fascia automatically. However, this is not the case with all programs, nor does it apply to all types of fascial tissue. Moreover, the

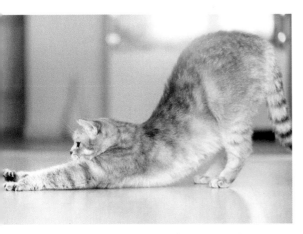

Cats instinctively use tensile stress to activate their muscles and fascia. This is not passive stretching, but active stretching that involves muscle contraction.

muscle fascia needs to be stimulated in certain ways in order to regenerate and remain energetic. Many popular training programs are geared primarily towards increasing strength, with little consideration given to the range of possibilities of human movement, and the different types and tasks of the fascial tissue in the body. The particular impulses that fascia and tendons need, especially for rebuilding, regeneration or fluid exchange, cannot simply be achieved by lifting weights or performing unilateral exercises. Intense weight training actually stimulates collagen production in fascia. The connective tissue cells increase their capacity because a strong muscle also requires a stronger fascia for its growth. This means an increase in the proportion of solid collagen fibres, which can limit mobility, especially when

performing unilateral physical exercises without any balance component. This can be seen in competitive athletes, such as the Tour de France riders: they intensively train their calf muscles and hamstrings, but then become stiff in the hips. For many athletes such as dancers, gymnasts, wrestlers and other sportspeople, it is important to have good mobility in the whole body. They need strength, flexibility and good all-round coordination. Because they protect against injury and enable us to carry out normal activities easily, mobility and good coordination should be the goal for those of us who aren't athletes, too.

How to access the fascia while training

As studies have shown, strength training and normal workout exercises do not necessarily train the fascia, too. This is partially due to the arrangement of the fibres in the fascia compared with that of the muscles. Fascia is structured as plates or sheaths around the different muscles, and their fibres run in different directions:

▶ parallel to the direction of the muscle
▶ transversely to the direction of the muscle, and
▶ in the direction of the muscle – i.e. fibres that run parallel to the front and back of the muscle, such as the tendons which attach the muscle to the bone.

Not an automatic process: muscle and fascia training

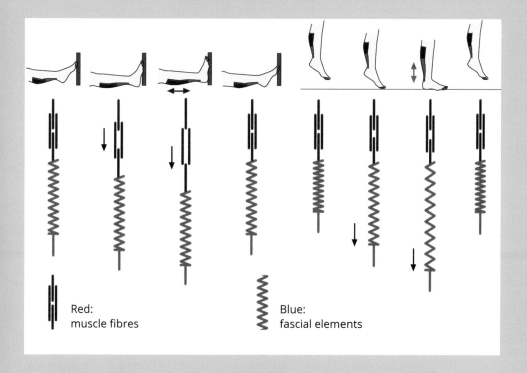

Red:
muscle fibres

Blue:
fascial elements

Left four illustrations: Here, the calf muscles are being trained using conventional exercises. The subject is pushing a plate away from them using their feet, which is a classic strength exercise. The red elements in the diagram represent the muscle fibres, which change in length during the exercise. The blue springs represent the elastic fascial structures. They undergo only very minor changes in length, and therefore remain largely unstimulated by this exercise.

The right four illustrations are different. Here, the exercise uses elastic suspension such as hopping or jumping actions. Now, the tendons – the blue fascial elements – also change in length, while the red muscle fibres hardly extend at all. In this case, it is the Achilles tendon that is being stimulated. When you hop, this moves up and down like a yo-yo, which is exactly the type of stimulation that it needs.

Stretching and training: what fascia needs

The images below show what happens to fascia when a muscle is subjected to various activities and stress. First, let's look at the inside of the muscle: the blue elements in the diagram represent fascia and fascial fibres that run in specific directions in and around the muscle.

Here we see the muscle and fascia fibres at rest: the fascial elements are arranged lengthways, transversely and serially to the muscle, as represented in blue. Like the red muscle tissue, all the fascial elements here are in a relaxed state.

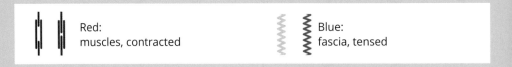

Red:
muscles, contracted

Blue:
fascia, tensed

In traditional strength exercises, the muscle changes state. Take a look at the blue elements in this example of the biceps muscle: if you hold a dumbbell in your hand and raise it so that the elbow bends, the biceps muscle contracts, shortens and widens. In the diagram, the muscle is seen to be bulging; this results in an elongation of the blue fascia elements which extend transversely. The tendon is under stress and contains the serially connected blue fascial fibres.

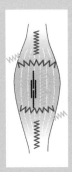

So far, so good. However, the fibres that run parallel to the muscle – the blue elements inside – are not accessed and do not get stretched. These are the perimysia and the endomysia – the sheaths of connective tissue around the muscle fibres. This fascia also needs to be stimulated if it is to metabolise and grow. This can be achieved using a combination of stretching and a particular type of muscle tension. We can see this effect in action in the following two illustrations:

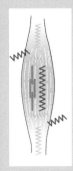

Passive expansion, as occurs in normal stretching. Here the muscle lengthens, but does not become thicker since it does not contract. As you can see, the pink elements are limp, but fascia that runs parallel to the muscle fibres is also elongated and tensed.

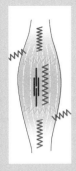

Tensile stress is what occurs when the muscle fibres are stretched and activated simultaneously. This is the case, for example, when a cat stretches while hooking its claws into the carpet. Now we see that both the red and blue elements change state: almost all parts of fascia are tensed and stimulated.

However, the fascial elements that run parallel to the muscle are not adequately stretched and stimulated during normal exercise or training. This applies in particular to popular sports like football, rounders, jogging, swimming and cycling.

By doing gentle stretches, we can reach deeper parts of the muscle and fascia than can be reached in strength-building exercises. These stretching exercises form an integral part of our training program, but we also include tensile stress – the combination of stretching and muscle contraction.

The exercises in our program incorporate all of these various effects of muscle strength, passive stretching and tensile stress. We have various different methods for doing this, all of which hone in on the fascial tissue arranged in various alignments in and around the muscle.

Features of healthy fascia and good fascia training

The goal of our fascia training is therefore to ensure that the fascia throughout our system is functioning at its best. From everything we have seen so far, we can assume that the characteristics of healthy, well-trained fascia are as follows:

1. It is firm and elastic at the same time.
2. It is flexible, a bit like bamboo.
3. It has the tensile strength of rope.
4. It allows us to make springing movements like those of a gazelle.

Fascia training:

▶ increases the resilience of our tendons and ligaments
▶ vprevents painful friction in the hip joints and intervertebral discs
▶ protects our muscles against injury
▶ keeps the body in shape by maintaining a youthful and toned profile.

There are clear advantages to having healthy fascia, for the way our bodies move when doing exercise and when going about our everyday lives:

▶ Our muscles work more efficiently.
▶ Recovery times are considerably shortened, so we recuperate faster for the next workout and the next task.

▶ Our performance increases. Our movement and coordination improve.
▶ Keeping our fascia in good condition can protect us against injury, pain and other disorders – well into old age.

Injuries, disorders, matting and adhesion of fascia are the common culprits behind many of the complaints and conditions from which we suffer, including lower back pain, shoulder pain, elbow problems, neck pain, the dreaded plantar fasciitis, and more. In all of these syndromes, the condition of the connective tissue plays an important role; in some instances, it may even be the root cause, such as in shoulder problems like frozen shoulder or in heel spurs. Most of the problems mentioned above are signs that our fascial network is responding in an obstructive way to being incorrectly exercised or underutilised.

What are we built for?

At some point, we have all marvelled in astonishment at the amazing feats achieved by circus acrobats, dancers, gymnasts, fencers, Judo fighters or extreme climbers on steep rock faces.

The human movement repertoire is extremely diverse; more so than in any other species of animal. We also belong to a species capable of consciously coordinating remarkably precise movements in tandem with other individuals – otherwise known as dancing! Descended from tree dwellers that pulled themselves from branch to branch, we later advanced to walking upright on two legs, developing into runners and dancers whose performance is characterised by economical endurance. It therefore stands to reason that natural movement for humans is marked by its extreme versatility. However, we do also have something in common with animals: our movements, and especially our ability to walk upright, defy two of the fundamental laws of physics, specifically those relating to gravity and the inertia of mass, which we have to overcome with every single movement we make. For my teacher Ida Rolf, the relationship between the body and gravity was an essential element around which she built her theory of body posture and movements.

We, like many animals, are built to contradict the force of gravity, but also to perform a broad spectrum of different movements. If one of or both of these elements is missing in our lives, our bodies respond with degeneration and illness. Without the stimulation they need, the muscles, bones and also the fascia begin to waste away, leading to pain and injury. Yet, our way of life in the Western world underutilises our bodies. We use only a tiny fraction of the broad range of movements of which our species is capable, and many of us do far too little exercise, especially as we age. Perhaps we feel that we can allow certain skills to quietly dwindle because we no longer need them in the modern world. However, the Stone Age still lingers in our bones! As the medical scientist Detlev Ganten of the Charité in Berlin intimates, we are truly suffering our loss. Our sore joints, slipped discs, arthritis and inflammation, not to mention obesity, metabolic disorders, diabetes and heart attacks are all symptoms of deficiency. They are our bodies' response to the inertia, underuse and unnatural strain that we inflict upon it. We mustn't forget that there are also serious psychological implications: there is evidence to show that depression, as well as several forms of dementia, are closely related to inactivity. We are becoming increasingly aware of the benefits of movement for our mental health.

You are no doubt well aware of these concerns about the implications of inactivity. However, aside from the importance of exercise in general, there is a growing awareness of how important the correct forms of movement are. Effective exercise regimes should include whole-body movements, with elements of coordination and dexterity, balance, stimulation of the long fascial lines, natural movement patterns and variation.

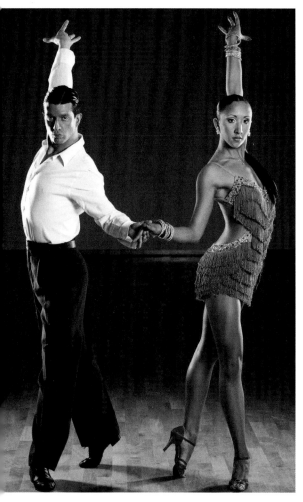

Extraordinary coordination: humans can coordinate their movements in exact tandem with one another.

do not use the full scope of movement of which our bodies are capable. Observations of apes have provided us with information about typical movement patterns: the animals hang, climb, jump, grip onto branches and support their own weight, squat, crawl and crouch – all the while moving, stretching and challenging their joints to the maximum.

Researchers propose that the reduced mobility associated with modern life – with people frequently sitting for long periods, wearing shoes and all the typical inactive lifestyles that come with city living – leads to illness because it restricts the natural scope of movement of our joints and we no longer stretch them as we should. This can lead to problems in the cartilage, such as arthritis in the fingers, which up to now has only been explained by excessive exposure to stress. So it seems it is actually the other way round, and that it is actually underuse rather than over-use that damages the joints, as well as not enough of the right kinds of movement.

Some researchers believe that only versatile, adequate demand on the musculoskeletal system guarantees health in the long term, as well as preventing arthritis and joint inflammation. This theory is what's known as the 'unused-arc' theory, and it refers to what happens when we

New Zealand-based anatomist Colin F. Alexander provides one example that supports this theory. He noticed that chimpanzees, in both their natural habitats and in modern zoos, are much less prone to degenerative joint diseases in old age than humans are – with one exception:

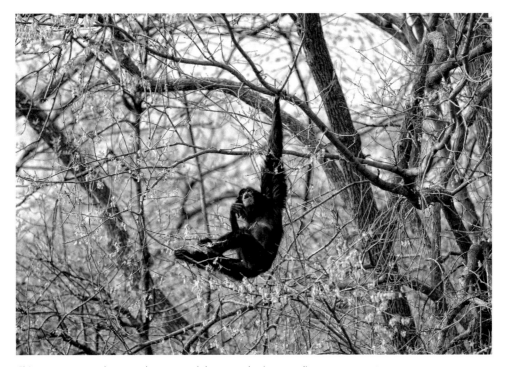

Chimpanzees move between the trees and the ground using very diverse movements.

chimpanzees kept in cages without adequate opportunities to climb and move in ways appropriate to their species display similar signs of ageing in their joints to those of humans. Could that be due to insufficient use of the range of movement in their joints? In order to investigate this theory, Alexander conducted a study of chimps, orangutans and humans, to see whether they use the full range of movement available to their joints while going about their day-to-day lives. The results showed that as long as they have the right living environment, monkeys use the full range of movement allowed by the anatomy of their joints. Humans, on the other hand, only use a small fraction of the possible scope of movement of their joints.

Here we have a clear correlation: the joints for which we utilise the full range of possible motion, such as the elbows, stay in good condition – like our monkey relatives. However, those joints for which we utilise only part of the spectrum of possible movement – such as the knees and hips – succumb to arthritic symptoms. The metabolic processes that take place in healthy connective tissue within these joints begin to stagnate, the layers of cartilage inside the joints become brittle and cracked, which in turn triggers repair processes. Then, instead of nice soft cartilage, we have bony tissue growing in the wrong places, which puts unnecessary pressure on the joint and causes pain.

As a general rule, the course of osteoarthritis would appear to support Alexander's theory. Osteoarthritis of the hip joint begins in the areas used the least, namely the edges, and then continues into the sites that are placed under more strain, such as the head of the femur. It is therefore possible that arthritis is not the result of wear and tear, but something quite different – the result of the under-use of our evolutionary system, or the result of not moving at all or not moving as we were made to do.

One consequence of these considerations is that doctors nowadays are far more likely to recommend movement, rather than rest, as a remedy to these problems. The success currently being seen in the use of climbing walls in hospitals and rehabilitation facilities also supports the unused-arc hypothesis.

Climbing activates our evolutionary spectrum of movement patterns and many muscles and ligaments simultaneously.

This requisite coordination also involves arms-over-the-head movements and the shoulder and neck muscles. This all yields great results in pain relief, back problems and recovery from spine surgery, and is also a successful aid to recovery in neurological domains, such as strokes, multiple sclerosis and anxiety disorders.

Aside from the context of clinics and illness, there is also a growing trend for everyday exercises and sports that match these findings, in the form of playgrounds for adults. These outdoor areas consist of climbing walls and adventure courses, where even the elderly can have a go and let off some steam. Not only are these activities a lot of fun, they are also very beneficial from a fascial perspective. I personally like to go to my local park in Munich as often as I can, where there is a climbing frame and a few monkey bars. I use these to practice all the possible monkey-like movements I can do, as you can see in the photo on page 21. After a long day in the laboratory or on the road, there is no better way to relax and rejuvenate. I believe that these sorts of playgrounds, where we can perform a diverse range of movements, are the key to the future of physical health. I will talk a little more about this from a fascial perspective at the end of this book (from page 283).

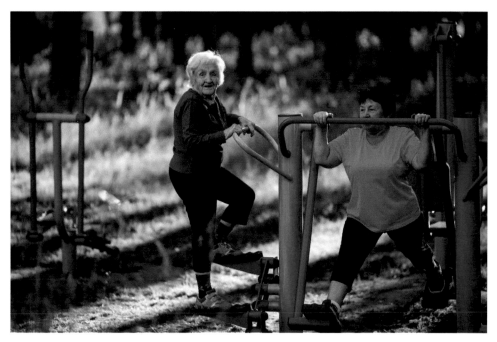

Pensioners on the playground: researchers are currently investigating the science behind the trend.

Move like a human

I have been fortunate enough to be able to exchange ideas on this exciting topic on several occasions with Dr Daniel Lieberman, one of the leading anthropologists of our time. Right at the beginning of his research career at Harvard University, Lieberman showed that it is the numerous fascial elements in human anatomy that prime us for movement, especially endurance running. This relates specifically to the plantar fascia, the neck fascia and the *fascia lata* on the outside of the thigh, which perfectly equip us to run long distances at a moderately high pace. What is really remarkable though,

is that we are better at it than almost all animals. Lieberman has drawn his own personal conclusions from this, in that he taught himself to jog barefoot and now promotes this activity as a healthy form of exercise that suits our species-specific needs – as do I. Of course, we can all agree that you can't just kick off your shoes and jog barefoot straight away. If you're not used to walking barefoot, you should start slowly and carefully, gradually building up your resilience at sensible intervals. If you ignore this crucial advice, you run the risk of painful overuse injuries such as heel spurs or inflammation in the plantar fascia and Achilles tendon.

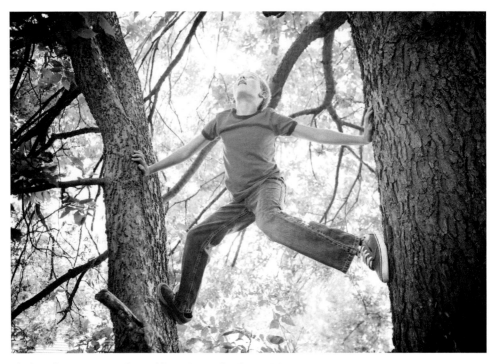

Climbing forces your muscles and fascia into unfamiliar positions.

After his research on running, Dr Lieberman devoted himself to another very typical human movement: throwing. This could also be described as an evolutionary development unique to humans, as we are the only species that can throw in a targeted way and at high speed. Again, Lieberman argued that the structure of the human shoulder is designed in such a way so as to enable fascial elements to store and discharge tensile energy as efficiently as possible. Humans can achieve enormous throwing speeds thanks to the particularly high elastic energy storage capacity of the fascia in our shoulders. Nowadays, adults in particular only really use these fascia in certain sports such as cricket or javelin, discus or hammer throwing. Children, on the other hand, perform the throwing action a lot more frequently. When they play with a ball or have a snowball fight, they are playfully practising this archaic motion for which humans were primed. Throwing was an essential component of human evolution, not only for hunting, but also earlier, when we would have had to deter rival tribes. It would definitely have been one of the targeted and coordinated movements that early humans are likely to have consciously practiced.

Lieberman's work on throwing has been extremely valuable to me personally. As an adult living life in the city, I would never have made time to practice this action – an action that is so intrinsic to our species – had it not been for the advice I received from him. I even suspect that many of the complaints relating to the shoulder and arm area from which so many people currently suffer are linked to our failure to perform those particular movements for which the shoulder was made: throwing, hanging and swinging from branch to branch. I have little doubt that many cases of painful shoulder stiffness, as well as tennis elbow and mouse arm syndrome, could be prevented if we were to frequently challenge our arms and shoulders in our day-to-day lives. Later on in the exercise chapter, we will show you a few exercises to help you do just that.

Lieberman did not stop there in his search for intrinsically human movements that we no longer use. Since 2015, he has been investigating two further movement patterns in the behaviour of our hunter-gatherer ancestors: carrying and digging. For our ancestors, carrying loads – children, food and building materials, for example – was a common part of everyday life, as was actively working the land in a bent-forward position. Nowadays, these activities are far less common within our range of day-to-day movements than in the past. To some

extent, they are even frowned upon, with dragging and bending often associated with low status and hard work. However, the anthropologist argues that these postures are intrinsically human and therefore belong to our evolutionary repertoire of movement. The lack of these movements could, according to Lieberman's ingenious theory, potentially lead to the degeneration of myofascial structures in the torso and hip area – both of which are common culprits in the back complaints of modern humans.

Lieberman's team is currently conducting research into this in Kenya and other regions, examining the thickness and strength of the fascia in the torsos of people who do lots of digging and carrying. The researchers are comparing this data with other people in Africa who do less manual labour, as well as with Western office workers. I, for one, am very curious to see what specific anatomical findings Lieberman's team will bring to light over the next few years. That said, we have already integrated some of his findings into our program, with the 'African bends' exercise. These are particularly good for the large lumbar fascia and help to prevent back pain. You can find the exercise on pages 162 and 163 in Chapter 3.

The pool of well-known experts in this field also includes German sports scientists

Ido Portal and the new theory of movement

Info

In recent years, innovative movement schools, such as the one run by Israeli Ido Portal, have become very popular. Portal is trained in Capoeira, the Brazilian martial art, and is also experienced in acrobatics, yoga and dance. His ethos is to promote general movement of the highest possible quality – according to him, people should strive to move in as versatile a way as possible. He also references evolution and the rich spectrum of natural movements that people are capable of and for which their bodies are adapted: running, dangling, crawling, rolling across the floor, climbing, jumping off things, scrambling and wresting with one another. Portal is all about diverse movements that use all the limbs – the types of movement that might be required by hunters and gatherers over the course of a day in the wild. Himself an exceptionally talented movement artist, Portal is opposed to the notion of early specialisation, such as encouraging children to focus on one sport for which they show particular prowess. He gives workshops all over the world, and if you want to see his impressive body coordination for yourself, you can find YouTube videos of him online.

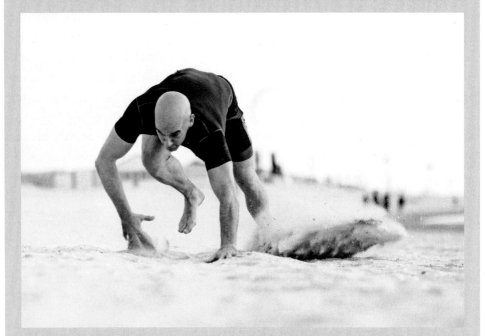

Humans are capable of a diverse range of natural movements.

Dr Kurt Mosetter and Edo Hemar. I also exchange ideas with them on a regular basis, and for the past few years, our discussions have intensified on the question of which are the most important and intrinsic movements for the human species. And what, then, do we need to do to keep our musculoskeletal system healthy in the long term? At the moment, I personally think that there are seven essential movements:

► running and walking
► climbing and swinging
► throwing,
► squatting
► carrying
► digging and other manual work that requires a bent posture
► dance and play.

Of course, this isn't to say that we should be heading 'back to the Stone Age', so to speak. However, it does makes sense to look specifically for ways to cultivate the sorts of movement patterns that early humans would have used. In today's world, these are missing from our day-to-day routines, and there is increasing evidence that our body needs them in order to stay healthy. Done properly, this should be the antidote to the common signs of degeneration in the joints, ligaments and bones. To practice these seven basic movements, I envisage having a playground specifically geared towards the physical capabilities of our species. It would be a bit like the outdoor gyms that already exist, but they would be expanded somewhat to include opportunities to practice the full range of movements, postures and actions in the human repertoire. If you were to visit such a playground, here's what you could do there:

► Short sprints, including hopscotch and a sort of obstacle course, plus a game of catch with frequent changes of direction.
► Dangling from one bar to the next and climbing (my favourite thing on the playground is what they call a space net – see the photo on page 21).
► Throwing, preferably against a wall; if necessary without letting go, as described in the exercise on page 207.
► Squatting (which usually happens automatically when there are no chairs nearby!).
► Weight-bearing exercises such as carrying loads on your head, giving someone a piggyback or a leg up, doing a shoulder stand.
► Stooping and bending, such as trying to move a heavy stone or pull out a root.
► Dance and play – ideally with music and other people, but put your competitive mindset to one side and focus on having fun!

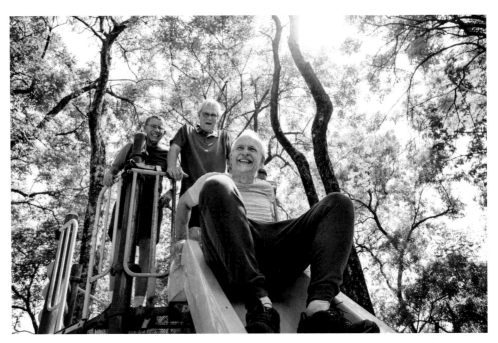

Exercise can be fun and enjoyable at any age, and the more fun you have, the more successful it will be!

The right stimuli for the fascial network

In light of these theories about species-appropriate movement and the functions of fascia, we can assume that, in order to exercise the connective tissue effectively, we need to combine a range of different training stimuli. We need a regime that challenges the various functions of our fascia and the entire network throughout the body, as well as one that helps to maintain the health and condition of the tissue. Fascia loves to be exercised and stretched, as well as having mechanical pressure and tension applied to it. Pressing or rolling out the fascia also encourages the exchange of fluids.

We will incorporate this into the training program, with exercises that include rolling out the tissue using a ball or specially prepared foam roller. This action achieves exactly the effect we're after: it squeezes out the fascia like a sponge. Our bodies then replace the lost fluid with new, fresh tissue fluid from the blood plasma in the tiny arteries nearby, thereby exchanging a decent proportion of the fluid in the ground substance. The pressing action acts as a kind of self-massage and can help with muscle pain and tension.

There is another important element to be considered: the stimulation of sensory functions in the fascia. As we now know from the first chapter, fascia can be regarded as our greatest sensory organ. Our movements are fundamentally dependent on the senses – the processing of sensory information from the muscles, joints and fascia. Activating and improving our sensory experience and interoceptive awareness are therefore essential components of fascia training. With regard to this aspect of the training, simply reeling off a rigid program of movements – 'going through the motions', so to speak – will not work. Focusing on our senses and genuinely feeling the movements will increase our enjoyment and sense of well-being. This, in turn, stimulates the release of important neurotransmitters in the brain such as dopamine. Dopamine affects our sense of happiness, motivation and even our ability to learn. It is closely linked with movement and enables us to learn and memorise the movements better. The reverse is also true, in that feelings of enjoyment, well-being and sensuality can also improve our sensory perception – and thus make the training more successful.

A brief summary

The training stimuli for exercising fascia include:

- ▶ variety of movement
- ▶ alternation between tensing and relaxing the muscles
- ▶ elastic suspension movements
- ▶ appropriate levels of tensile force to promote elastic storage capacity
- ▶ use of the functional units of fascial lines throughout the body
- ▶ activation of intrinsic patterns of movement
- ▶ maintenance and regeneration
- ▶ soft, steady stimulation, such as through stretching, stroking and massage
- ▶ sensory impulses and perception exercises.

The four dimensions of fascia training

Our fascia training therefore needs to be as diverse as possible and address the various functions of the fascial system. That's why our training program is built on four principles which correspond to the four basic functions of fascia that we looked at in Chapter 1 (page 33). For each of these four basic functions, there are targeted training stimuli. These make up the four dimensions of the fascia workout, as shown in the pie chart: stretch, spring, feel and revive. If you compare these dimensions to the basic functions, you can see that each basic function corresponds to one particular type of exercise:

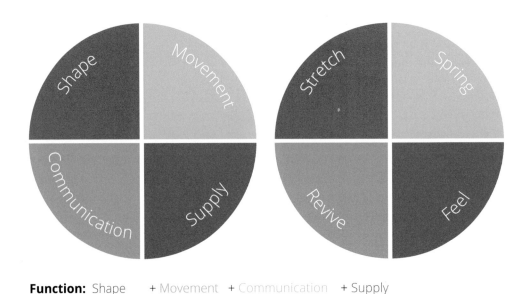

Function: Shape   + Movement + Communication + Supply
Training: Stretch   + Spring   + Revive   + Feel

It's no accident that we used a pie chart with a cross in the centre to represent these dimensions. The circle represents a continuum, referring to the holistic nature of the four functions. The cross in the centre represents the four different dimensions of the training dimensions – all of which are necessary in order to access the fascial tissue. They differ from each other and have to be considered individually. In spite of this, however, they do actually belong together and all four should be exercised in order to ensure that all types of fascial tissue are stimulated, including that in the deeper layers and the linked chains.

The circle with the cross will guide you through Chapter 3 and help to keep you on the right track. It shows you which exercise corresponds to which function, which complaints or problems needs to be addressed by which basic functions and what kind of training stimulus needs to be applied. For this purpose, the colour of each area matches the colour of the respective term. However, before we get started with the actual exercises, let's take a closer look at how the four dimensions of the workout address the four basic functions.

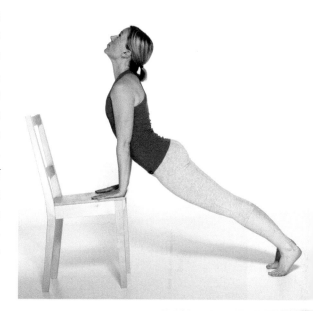

1. Stretch – basic function: Shape

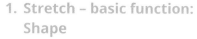

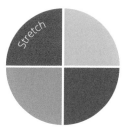

Stretching stimulates the mechanical qualities of fascia as the substance that gives the body shape. It is a natural form of strain that is applied in many kinds of movement – but conventional stretching in particular will activate the long fascial lines. Stretching exercises have been included in training programs for centuries, especially those designed for dancers and acrobats. Stretching can actually extend our range of motion, and this includes not only the muscles but the joints as well. However, it can also do a lot

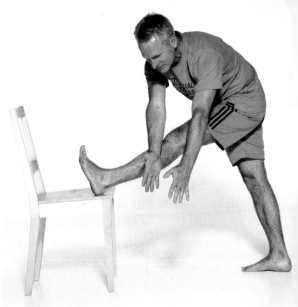

more, as only discovered through years of research. Yoga, which has experienced significant global success, is based on the stretching of fascial tissue. Slow, methodical stretches held for a long duration have

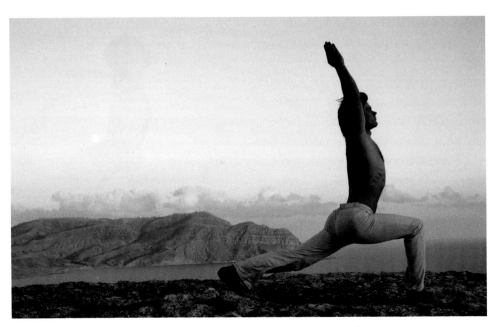

Yoga affects fascia. Research has recently begun into the connections between the two.

significant physiological effects, reducing blood pressure and lowering your heart rate. That is because, when fascial tissue is stretched, signals are transmitted to the autonomic nervous system. This reduces activity levels in the system responsible for stress – the sympathetic nervous system – which indirectly causes the body to relax. This is essentially the science behind the mysterious effects of meditative yoga and its ability to bring a sense of calm to our stressed-out minds.

However, it does more than calm us down. Animal studies have shown that yoga-style stretching actually alleviates pain, such as in rats with inflammation in their backs. Moreover, yoga has since been scientifically proven to help ease back pain in humans, too. The crucial factor here is stretching. An American study showed that back pain patients who did yoga-style stretching exercises achieved results that were as good as those for patients who completed a conventional back training program. This, in turn, has strengthened the reputation of yoga, which is now accepted by health insurance companies as a remedy for back ache and many other complaints. You can read more about this, as well as details on the studies and the new Yin style of yoga, in Chapter 4.

Caught in the scientific crossfire: stretching trends from 1985 to the present day	
Then: 1985 to 2015	**Now**
Springing movements when stretching are outdated, inefficient and dangerous.	Springing stretches are back in fashion, especially for training the elasticity of fascia.
Slow, gentle stretches work best.	Stretching while actively straining the muscle, as well as stretching while doing small, rocking jumps, can be just as beneficial as slow, gentle stretching.
Stretching before exercise is very important and highly recommended because it lowers the risk of injury.	It is unclear whether static stretching will reduce the risk of injury. In fact, it may even increase it! Stretching just before exercise can definitely reduce the explosive take-off power of athletes in sports such as sprinting, handball and basketball, where a high degree of elasticity is needed. Static stretching immediately before a game or race will mean you cannot jump as high or sprint as quickly.
Stretching after exercise speeds up the regeneration process.	Stretching after exercise has little to no effect on the regeneration process.
When stretching, it is important to relax the stretched muscle as much as possible.	On the contrary: It is beneficial to contract the muscle at regular intervals against an external resistance. This not only enables the stretch to access the intramuscular connective tissue, but also the tendon connected to the muscle.
It is important to stretch each specific muscle group individually. It is best to stretch each muscle in turn, one after the other.	It is important to also stretch the long fascial lines that stretch across multiple joints; not just individual muscles.
When stretching, it is important to adopt and hold the 'correct' stretching position, making it as accurate as possible.	On the contrary: It is important to alternate between different angles as you stretch, pulling in different directions in order to reach the different parts of fascia. It works best to make it as varied as possible.
Stretching only benefits the musculoskeletal system.	Stretching for several minutes also has other physiological effects: it relaxes the body, reduces chronic inflammation and promotes wound healing. It can be used for these specific objectives.

However, stretching has been caught in the crossfire between different theories of modern sports science since the 1980s. There are different types of stretching, including dynamic, bobbing stretches – such as trying to touch your toes with your fingertips, while bouncing your heels in short bursts – as well as slow, static stretches that are held for longer. The latter involves carefully assuming a stretching pose and holding it for a longer period, without teetering. The bouncing stretches, although practiced for centuries by gymnasts and dancers, fell into disrepute among some sports scientists, who felt they had no real benefits and were prone to causing injury. This happened in the 1980s, when slow stretching became a popular warm-up for exercise. The idea was that it warmed up the muscle and protected it from injury, although this theory has never been proven. Later, the advocates of slow, static stretching as the ultimate warm-up had some back-pedalling to do. Now, dynamic bouncing stretches have been fully resurrected, even within the sports science community.

When it comes to training fascia, we use both forms of stretching: dynamic bouncing to and fro in a stretch pose, as well as slow, static stretching. They each serve a different purpose and support different physiological types of connective tissue. We consider it ineffective to exclusively stretch out isolated, individual muscles. The exercises in our program therefore take the form of a playful, creative full-body workout, with stretches for both the muscles and the fascia. These simple exercises include versions of some well-known stretching exercises, which we have tweaked slightly in order to stimulate the whole musculofascial system.

2. Spring, basic function: Movement

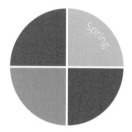

Suspension or 'springing' exercises, such as hopping or swinging the upper body, stimulate the elastic storage capacity of fascia, which is important for basic movement functions. This applies to all muscle fibres, but especially to the tendons. The principle of tensile energy features in all exercises of this kind, as they involve elastic recoil movements.

One variant is pre-loading, which involves a slight counter-movement in which the tendons and fascia are charged with energy, similarly to when a javelin thrower extends their arm backwards in preparation for the throw. Pre-loading plays a significant role, especially in our day-to-day

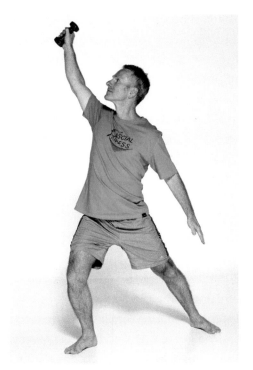
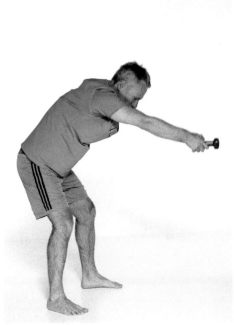

movements. Bending over and coming up again, for example, as well as lifting objects both light and heavy, involve pre-loading of the fascia. Springing exercises that use the whole body also stimulate the long fascial lines. You can do them in all different directions to make sure you stimulate all the different fascial lines.

Take care to ensure that it is actually a springing motion, rather than a swinging motion like that of a pendulum. They look similar from the outside, but they differ in terms of whether or not they use the elastic storage capacity of fascia itself, or whether the kinetic energy is transferred via the gravitational force and swinging

motion. For example, if you were to hold a bucket in your hand and swing it rhythmically back and forth, you would barely use the elastic storage capacity of fascia. That is because, in this movement, the momentum is created by gravity – specifically, by the difference in height between the highest and lowest point of the swinging curve. It works differently when you perform dynamic suspensions. Here, fascia stretches to the end of the arc of the motion and then snaps back again, such as when you hop up and down. In this case, the kinetic energy is briefly stored in the Achilles tendon and other sections of fascia in the leg. Then, the stretched fibres spring back and the stored energy is discharged – like releasing a catapult.

When we do our training, the acceleration phase should be very short – around 0.2 to 0.3 seconds. If it were to last a whole second or even longer, we might produce a lovely movement, but it would not train fascia. This can be illustrated using the example of a squat: squatting every two seconds will work the muscles in the buttocks and thighs, but not the large fascial lines in those areas. The only way to work this tissue is to bounce your knees while standing, keeping up a fast rhythm. That is what makes it a 'fascial movement', so to speak, because it briefly tenses fascia in the thighs, which then snaps back to its original shape. This does not happen when you bend your knees in a squatting position.

3. Revive, basic function: Supply

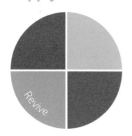

For the part of the program designed to revive and rejuvenate fascia, we propose a kind of self-massage. To do this, we use foam rollers, which are available from

sports shops. In some cases, you can use a tennis ball or rubber ball as an alternative, but please follow the guidance on page 133 of Chapter 3.

In all these exercises, pressure is applied to the connective tissue as it would be during a massage. This triggers a purely mechanical process of fluid exchange in fascia. The tissue is literally wrung out like a sponge, pushing out metabolic waste and lymph, and then refills itself with fresh fluid. The squeezed out tissue sucks in fresh fluid, although a certain amount of the old fluid also seeps back in. The fresh fluid comes from the blood plasma in the tiny blood vessels nearby. While the drained fluid contains harmful metabolic waste products – and sometimes inflammatory neurotransmitters – the fluid newly drawn in from the plasma is clean and fresh. This is what enables the renewal process to happen in fascia.

It is therefore beneficial to squeeze out the sponge-like tissue not just once, but several times, pushing the fluid in different directions. Some therapists advise that such rolling movements should only be carried out in the direction of the lymphatic vessels, i.e. towards the trunk of the body. It is certainly the case that this is beneficial if the subject has a pronounced lymphatic disorder, such as lymphedema. However, 90 percent of the fluid from the

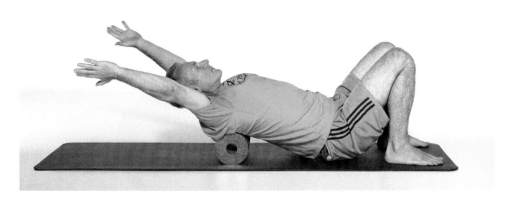

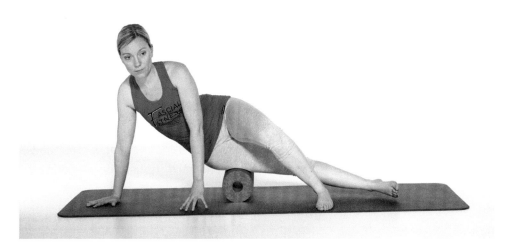

connective tissue and the ground substance is drained off through small veins that run in various different directions, and not through the lymphatic system. We therefore recommend that you roll the tissue in a variety of directions when you do your training. This is the best way to support the renewal of the fluid in the tissue. You can find more about this in Chapter 3 on page 144 and page 158, as well as in Chapter 4.

This sort of fluid exchange stimulates the metabolism and improves the supply to fascia, but also to the associated organs. This is why we put pressure-based exercises for regenerating and rejuvenating fascia in the 'Supply' category. This effect can also be achieved with various methods of manual physiotherapy. Fascia loves pressure, and especially the right level of sliding pressure described above, as if you were squeezing out a sponge. It reacts particularly well to the application of this persistent, slow, gentle pressure. These are the sorts of techniques we use in Rolfing therapy, and treatments such as myofascial release and osteopathic grips also use the same effect. As we found out in Chapter 1, pressure also triggers a cascade of signals to be sent via the mechanoreceptors to the autonomic nervous system and in the direction of our muscles. This has a variety of effects. For example, appropriately applied pressure can reduce tautness in the fascia and muscle, releasing tension and adhesions in the tissue.

The 'revive' exercises in our fascia workout – which include elements of massage – are designed to regenerate the tissue, promoting a greater sense of body awareness and significantly improving our flexibility. The exercises that use a foam roller can be used as part of a daily exercise routine, but you can also use them at any time as a quick self-treatment to release tension and alleviate pain and soreness. There is now a sizeable market for pressure-based fascial treatments, such as self-massage, trigger point treatment, BLACKROLL training, and many more. We will talk more about this, as well as giving an overview of the latest fascia trends, in Chapter 4.

4. Feel, basic function: Communication

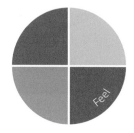

Feeling and noticing our movements is extremely important for our physical mobility and for the brain, as we discussed in Chapter 1. In kinesiology and scientific training, but also in psychology, this body perception and body self-image are now considered to be fundamentally important. This internal awareness of our body's movements is also gaining in importance with regard to increasing levels of inactivity in our modern-day lives. Clearly, it also plays a major role in many neurological and also psychological illnesses. In recent years, there has been a lot of research into the concept of 'embodiment'.

'Embodiment' is the word used by today's psychologists to describe the close correlation between physical changes in the body and our mental well-being. Many new and important findings have now

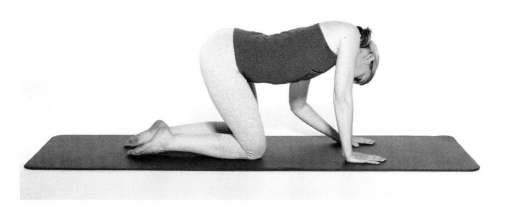

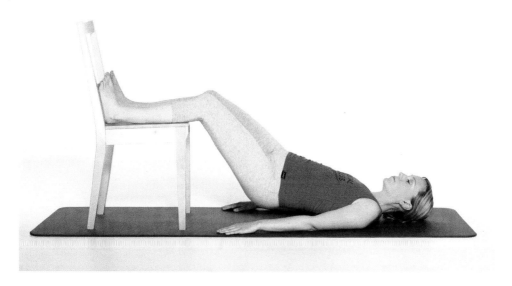

been collected in this field. For example, we now know that our posture not only affects how we perceive ourselves, but also how we view the world around us. Conversely, our emotional experiences trigger changes to our physical tension, as well as lasting biochemical responses – releasing hormones and

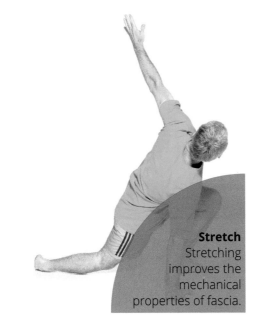
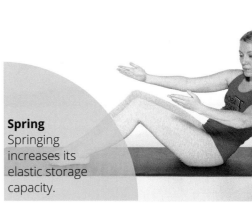

Stretch
Stretching improves the mechanical properties of fascia.

Spring
Springing increases its elastic storage capacity.

The principles of the workout

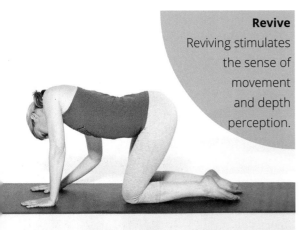
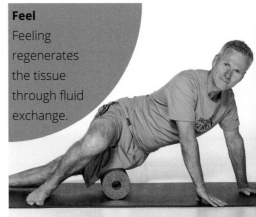

Revive
Reviving stimulates the sense of movement and depth perception.

Feel
Feeling regenerates the tissue through fluid exchange.

neurotransmitters and activating certain control circuits within our nervous system. One of the most recent findings, which is of particular interest, is that people who have a poorer perception of their own moods and feelings than others experience more pain and other physical symptoms with no apparent organic cause. Conversely, people with poor physical self-awareness are more prone to psychological disorders such as anxiety and depression.

In the fascia workout, we use sensory stimuli and perception exercises to strengthen our sense of feeling and increase body awareness. Small movements and subtle changes in the location or direction on which you are focused should help you to enjoy and explore your own movements. This sense of feeling or noticing occurs in a variety of exercises. The idea is to have fun and enjoy a playful exploration of your body. Think of it as a musical instrument that you can use to play all sorts of wonderful music! All this will tap into your fascia and thereby sharpen your awareness of movement and coordination, improving your overall agility and fitness. The important thing is to try not to get distracted during practice, and stay connected to your body. Only then will there be a benefit that registers in your brain, which is also how the training effects real change in your body.

Before we begin: which tissue type are you?

After discussing all the theory and many principles, I am sure you will be eager to finally get started. To begin, I invite you to take this short test to work out which type of connective tissue you have. This test will be useful because there is a whole spectrum of naturally occurring types of connective tissue. At either end of this spectrum, we have two poles: at one end, we have people with loose, soft connective tissue, who we call 'contortionists'; at the other, we have people with tight, firm connective tissue, who we call 'Vikings'.

People tend to be born into one of these two types. In other words, we enter the world with a genetic predisposition towards a certain tissue type, although this can also be influenced by other external factors over the course of our lives.

▶ Contortionists have soft connective tissue, tend to be highly flexible and therefore have low joint stability.
▶ Vikings have firm connective tissue, tend to have low flexibility and high stability, and are more prone to scar formation.

There is a third type, which is characterised by a specific combination of stiff and weak areas. This is known as the cross-over type. This type is especially common in modern industrial countries, where most people fall into this type. All three types are completely normal. Contortionists and Viking types occur with about the same frequency, while the majority of people are crossover types.

The pattern of strong and weak areas in crossover types is always the same and is not to be confused with the mixed type, which falls in the middle of the spectrum.

Crossover type
▶ **Stiff and shortened:** neck, upper chest, back extensors, lumbar fascia, back of the upper thighs and calves.
▶ **Weak and loose:** front neck area, shoulder stabilisers, abdomen, gluteus maximus.

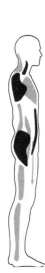

Because there are more crossover types than there are Vikings or contortionists, physiotherapists and doctors – as well as sports coaches – deal with this pattern a lot. We will come back to this later when we look at the exercises.

There are more male Vikings than female, as women tend to fall into the types with soft connective tissue. This tendency is due to physiological differences between the sexes:

▶ Men have more muscle mass and stronger muscles, and so their fascia is also stronger.
▶ In men, subcutaneous fat tends to be more tightly bound than in women.
▶ Women have a somewhat looser connective tissue structure, because the fascial tissue has to change during pregnancy and birth, with the pelvis expanding to make room for the baby.
▶ Women store different types of fat – and more of it – in the subcutaneous layers than men do. This is a natural mechanism that acts as a reserve for pregnancy and breastfeeding.

However, there are also women with firmer connective tissue – female Vikings, so to speak. There are also some very flexible men who would fall into the contortionist category. We know from everyday experience that, most of the time, it becomes apparent during childhood who is 'flexible' and who isn't. Girls and boys who are naturally flexible can do the splits fairly easily, whereas those who are less flexible have to practice and may never succeed.

Unlike Vikings and contortionists, the crossover type is not genetically predetermined. With this type, the stiff spots and weak areas develop over the course

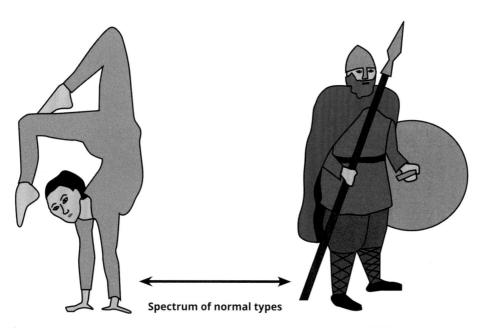

Spectrum of normal types

The natural scale ranges from hypermobile contortionists and dancers to stable, stiff Viking types.

of the individual's life, as a result of predominant use of one side of the body. Crossover types therefore tend to fall closer to the contortionist end or the Viking end of the spectrum from birth, but then the typical crossover pattern of stiffness and weakness gradually arises as they age.

Ballerinas, acrobats and gymnasts mostly belong to the flexible type, although they also need a lot of muscle power. Male Viking types are less likely to excel in these sports, because dancers, gymnasts and acrobats need to be flexible. The entire spectrum is a natural continuum, with some individuals falling relatively close to one extreme, while others fall more in the middle. Each of these connective tissue types come with their own typical sets of physical complaints. People with soft connective tissue are more prone to cellulite, herniated discs and stretch marks after pregnancy.

The firmer types, who we call Vikings, are more prone to scarring and to a condition we call 'Viking disease'. This causes fascia in the hands to stiffen, contract and form tight strings. This can be so extreme that the fingers become deformed. It often affects older men. This syndrome is particularly widespread in regions where Scandinavians settled during the

Contortionists

Info

Contortionists train their hypermobility from childhood; in particular, they increase the range of motion of their joints and systematically stretch their connective tissues.

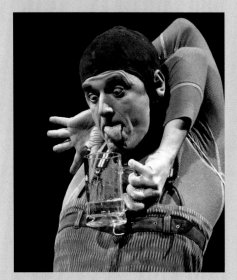

The contortionist and comedian Barto.

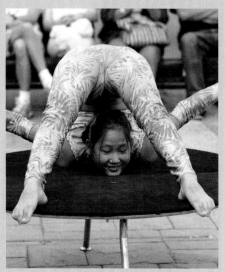

The young Mongolian contortionist Enkhmurum commenced her training at the age of six.

Thanks to this type of training, they are extremely agile and can contort their bodies into extraordinary positions. These incredible artists still perform in circuses today. Traditionally, they would be trained in Eastern circus schools, especially in Asia. Many of the acrobats are women, although there are some men, too. Contortionists are inherently more mobile than other people, but that is not to say that they suffer from pathological hypermobility, as is the case with Marfan syndrome or Ehlers-Danlos syndrome, which are caused by congenital defects in the connective tissue.

Migration Period, hence the name 'Viking disease'.

This condition belongs to a group of disorders of the connective tissue called fibromatoses. It can be uncomfortable, but it is benign. The symptoms are caused by inefficient collagen synthesis in fascia, whereby the myofibroblasts – the special contractile cells in the connective tissue – become overactive. Men are two-to-eight times more likely to be affected than women. Viking types have more shoulder problems such as stiffness or frozen shoulder. Parallel to the hand syndrome mentioned above, Viking types are also more prone to developing nodes and hard lumps in the connective tissue in their feet, the medical name for which is plantar fibromatosis. As you can see, the advantages and disadvantages of those types at either end of the spectrum are quite evenly distributed.

Crossover types have their own set of problems. They are more prone to pain in the neck and lumbar spine, as they tend to suffer from high levels of tension in these areas. On the other hand, they are also prone to having a chronic hollow back, which can actually be an advantage in certain sports, such as dancing or short-distance sprinting. Our aim is therefore not to eradicate or 'train away' all the manifestations of this pattern.

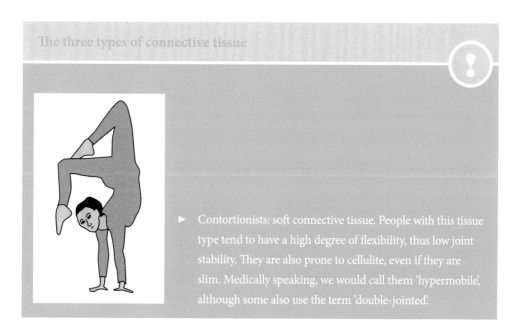

The three types of connective tissue

► Contortionists: soft connective tissue. People with this tissue type tend to have a high degree of flexibility, thus low joint stability. They are also prone to cellulite, even if they are slim. Medically speaking, we would call them 'hypermobile', although some also use the term 'double-jointed'.

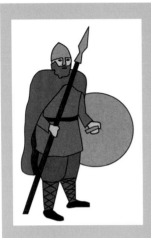

▶ **Vikings:** firm connective tissue. People with this tissue type tend to be less flexible but with a high degree of stability. They are more prone to scarring and often have attached earlobes. Medically speaking, we would call them 'hypomobile'.

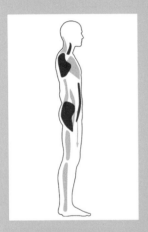

▶ **Crossover types:** characteristic combination of tight, stiff tissue in some areas and weak tissue in others. People with this tissue type are prone to stiffness in the neck, chest muscles, back, lumbar fascia, hip joints and the back of the legs. Typical weak points include: the shoulder blades, gluteus maximus, the front of the neck and the abdomen.

People with these three tissue types – Vikings, contortionists and crossover types – will benefit from different variations of the exercises. In the exercise chapter on page 191, you will therefore find a different set of guidelines for each of the three types.

You can use the tests on page 120 to work out which tissue type you have, and we highly recommend that you do. It will change how you see yourself, help you to understand why you experience certain symptoms and, ultimately, it will help you to pick the right exercises and get the most out of your fascia training. Start with Test A, which is for everyone. That will tell you if you are a contortionist type, in which case you can stop there. That's one end of the scale. If you only score a few points on this test, however, you should move on to the Viking test. Depending on your results, you may then answer the questions for the crossover type. You will find guidance for this in the test process and the results.

Of course, some people will differ slightly from the descriptions of each type or they may be a mixture of all three, but – generally speaking – we all fall into one of the three categories. You can do all of the tests at home wearing thin gym clothes and with bare feet, simply on the carpet or on a yoga mat.

Please note: All of the tests are designed for men and women – there are no separate tests. Both sexes can fall into any of the three types.

Important note

▶ All of these tests are practical tests used by medical professionals. They are based on a set of diagnostic criteria for determining an individual's genetic predisposition or for diagnosing certain diseases, which also includes what is known as the 'Beighton Score' and incorporates the findings of the Czech neurologist Vladimir Janda. He was particularly concerned with imbalances and disorders of the muscles and connective tissue. For example: the crossover type, as we call it here, is also known as the 'Janda type'.

▶ It is important to remember that the different connective tissue types and the results of the self-test have nothing to do with illness or pathology. They are just different manifestations of health. These tests therefore do not provide a medical diagnosis.

▶ The test questions and results are based on general day-to-day movements. People with actual connective tissue disorders need to be examined more closely. If you suspect that you have a connective tissue disorder or illness – because you often experience pain and injuries, for example – then please see a specialist before you start the fascia training.

Tests to determine types of connective tissue

Contortionists – the flexible type

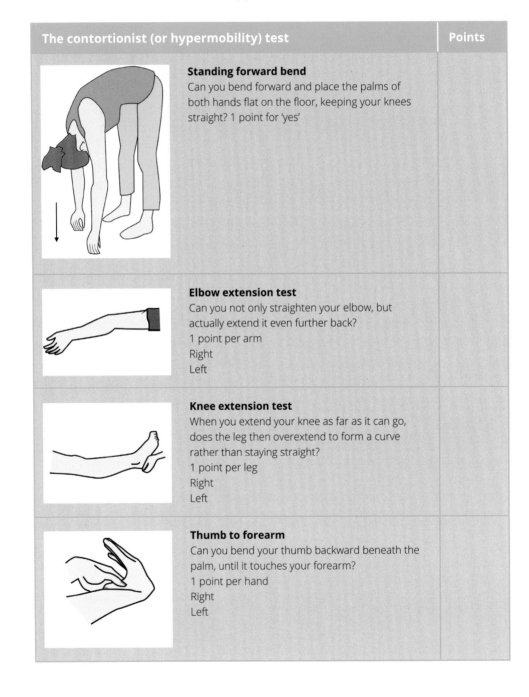

The contortionist (or hypermobility) test	Points
Standing forward bend Can you bend forward and place the palms of both hands flat on the floor, keeping your knees straight? 1 point for 'yes'	
Elbow extension test Can you not only straighten your elbow, but actually extend it even further back? 1 point per arm Right Left	
Knee extension test When you extend your knee as far as it can go, does the leg then overextend to form a curve rather than staying straight? 1 point per leg Right Left	
Thumb to forearm Can you bend your thumb backward beneath the palm, until it touches your forearm? 1 point per hand Right Left	

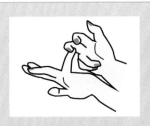

Little finger extension test
Can you bend your little finger more than
90 degrees backward, in the direction of your
forearm?
1 point per hand
Right
Left

Max. 9 points in total

Evaluation

6 or more points: Physically, it is highly likely that you are a contortionist type, which means your connective tissue is soft and supple. We may even say that people of this type have the 'gift of flexibility'.

4 or 5 points: It is not clear which tissue type you belong to from these test results alone. However, there are a few indications that would suggest you are genetically predisposed towards a softer connective tissue type. If you answer 'yes' to at least two of the following statements, you can assume that you are a contortionist type:

▶ Do you have detached earlobes?
▶ Is your frenulum – the fold of tissue beneath your tongue – thin and flexible?
▶ Do you bruise easily?
▶ Did you develop spinal curvature – also known as scoliosis – during puberty?

▶ Do you find that your wounds take a long time to heal?
▶ Do your joints easily dislocate on a day-to-day basis?

If you answered 'yes' to fewer than two of these questions, or if you are unsure which ones apply to you, please now take the Viking test.

0 to 3 points: You have no genetic disposition towards general hypermobility. Move on to the next test to see if you are a Viking type.

Contortionist types often find that they have relatively poor proprioceptive awareness in their joints. That means that the brain does not receive adequate signals of the kind that help to control movement and force. In the exercise chapter, you will find advice aimed specifically towards contortionist types, which should help to improve the proprioception in your joints.

Vikings – the robust type

The Viking (or hypomobility) test	VP (Viking points)
If you scored fewer than 3 points in the contortionist test, then you automatically score 3 Viking points (VP).	
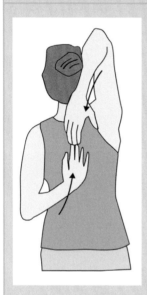 **Hands behind your back** If you try to bring your hands together behind your back – either with the right hand above or below the left – but you cannot get your hands closer than one hand-length apart, give yourself 1 VP.	
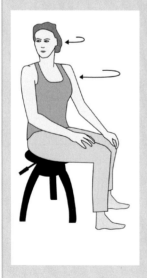 **Seated torso rotation** Sit on a chair, without leaning on the backrest. Turn your upper body and head to the right as far as you can, and then to the left, without moving your pelvis and legs. If you cannot turn in either direction so that the tip of your nose is at 90 degrees, give yourself 1 VP.	

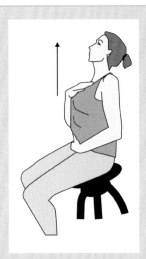

Seated torso stretch test

Sit up straight on a chair without leaning on the backrest. Place one hand on your lower abdomen, with your thumb in front of the navel, and the other hand on your sternum. Now, without moving your lower abdomen or the hand you have placed there, try to stretch your sternum and your top hand upwards and away from your bottom hand as far as possible. As you do this, feel free to shuffle and stretch your whole upper body upwards.

If you cannot stretch high enough to get your top hand at least one hand-width away from the bottom, give yourself 1 VP.

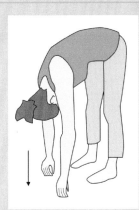

Forward bend

From a standing position, bend forward and try to touch the floor with your fingertips. If the distance between your fingertips and the floor is one hand-length or more, give yourself 1 VP.

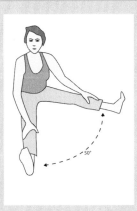

Straddle test

Sit on the floor in a straddle position. If you cannot get your legs more than 50 degrees apart, give yourself 1 VP.

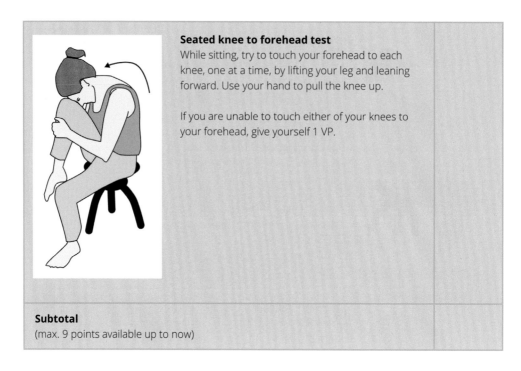

Seated knee to forehead test
While sitting, try to touch your forehead to each knee, one at a time, by lifting your leg and leaning forward. Use your hand to pull the knee up.

If you are unable to touch either of your knees to your forehead, give yourself 1 VP.

Subtotal
(max. 9 points available up to now)

Additional factors for calculating your Viking points

Use the following table to deduct points from your subtotal, according to your age and sex. Please select only one option.

Male and over 35: deduct 2 points	
Male and 35 or younger: deduct 1 point	
Female and over 35: deduct 1 point	
Female and 35 or older: points remain the same	
Total number of points:	

Evaluation

5 to 9 points: It is likely that you are a Viking type, which means the structure of your connective tissue is relatively firm. We may even say that people of this type have the 'gift of stability'.

3 to 4 points: You have some limitations in your movement and are closer to the Viking end of the spectrum, but it is not 100% clear from this test whether your genetic constitution falls into the Viking category. It is likely that your fitness level and lifestyle play as big a part in your ten-dency towards stability or hypomobility as your genetic make-up. Please move on to the next test – the crossover test. This will help you to determine whether your pro-file fits more with the crossover type.

Fewer than 3 points: You only have local-ised stiffness, but your general physiology does not fit that of a Viking type. Along our spectrum, you fall somewhere in the 'nor-mal' range of people with average mobil-ity. However, it is also quite possible that you are a crossover type. Continue to the next test.

The crossover type

Typical combination of stiffness and weak areas

Crossover types have a particular combination of stiff and weak areas in the body. The pattern is always the same and therefore differs from the spectrum of mixed types that fall between contortionists and Vikings. By the time you have finished this test, you will know whether you fall more into the category of mixed types or crossover types. The tips in the exercises on Chapter 3 are geared towards contortionists in terms of building up weak areas, and Vikings in terms of alleviating stiffness.

The crossover type test	Points
▶ Each time the restricted movement described applies to you, give yourself 2 points. ▶ Each time it applies to you, but only generally speaking, give yourself 1 point. ▶ If it absolutely does not apply to you, give yourself 0 points.	
Chin to chest While standing, bend your head down, keeping your mouth closed, and try to touch your sternum with your chin. If you can only bend so far that you can fit two or more fingers between your chin and your sternum, give yourself 2 points.	

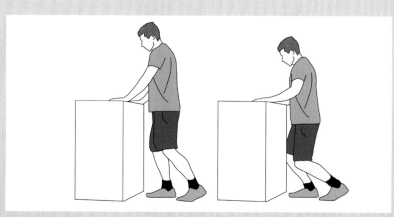

Knee to wall test

Stand in front of a wall, placing your hands against it at shoulder height to support your weight. Push one foot forward until the tip of your toe touches the wall. Then, with the same leg, bend the knee until it touches the wall.

Then pull your foot back an inch or two and try again to touch your knee against the wall. If you cannot move your foot further than 10 cm from the wall without becoming unable to touch your knee against the wall, give yourself 2 points.

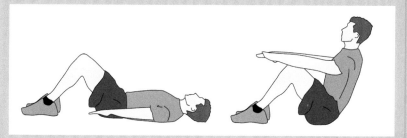

Sit-up test

Lie on your back with your legs bent. Shuffle your feet up until they are about two foot-lengths from your buttocks. Lay your head down and stretch out your arms to an angle of about 45 degrees to your body, resting them on the floor.
Now try to sit up as you would with a classic sit-up exercise, pulling your upper body up without moving your feet or lifting them off the floor. Your feet must stay in constant contact with the floor as you sit up. Try to come into a seated position with your upper body straight.

If you cannot sit up or you can only sit up by moving your feet, give yourself 2 points.

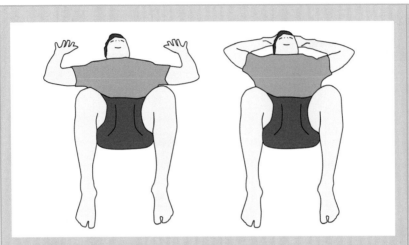

Fallen angel

Lie on your back and bend both of your elbows and upper arms at right angles, bringing them to shoulder level. Your bent arms should be resting on the floor, with your hands pointing straight upwards – parallel to your head. Then, without changing the angle of your elbows, try to move your upper arms further up towards your head, keeping them on the floor.

Go as far as you can without your elbows lifting up off the floor. If you cannot move either of your upper arms any further than 45 degrees to the side of your head, give yourself 2 points.

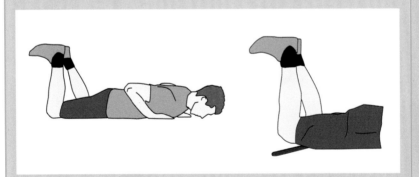

Hip stretch

We also call this test the 'lying skydiver'. Lie down on your stomach. Then lift one leg at a time, with your knee bent. As you raise each leg, use one hand to feel at what point a noticeable hollow forms in the small of your back. If you cannot lift either of your knees more than a hand's length from the floor without a hollow forming in your back, give yourself 2 points.

Total (max. 10 points)

Evaluation

6 to 10 points: You clearly demonstrate the pattern of weak areas and stiffer areas that is typical of the crossover type.

4 to 6 points: You have a tendency towards the crossover constellation, but the results are not conclusive.

0 to 2 points: You are not a true crossover type.

If you scored 6 points or more in this test, you can consider yourself a crossover type. If you don't seem to fit into any of the three typologies, then may we congratulate you on being truly unique! You are probably one of those people who is neither particularly mobile nor immobile, or perhaps just hold a bit of tension in certain areas. Of course, there is still every reason to train your fascia. You will work out for yourself which of the exercises in Chapter 3 best suit your needs.

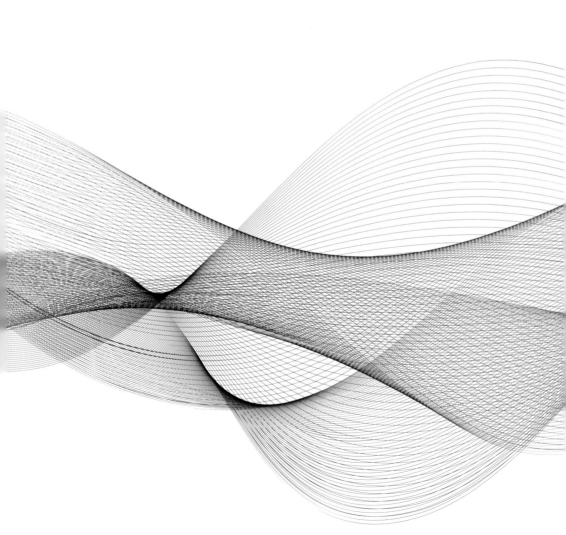

Chapter 3

The exercises

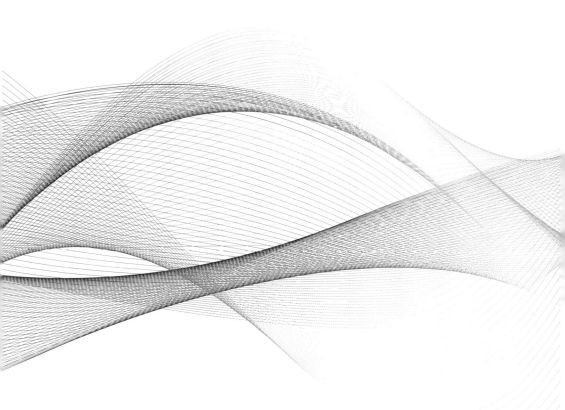

A tlast – the exercises! Now that you have battled through the long chapter on theory, it is time for the practice. Our fascial fitness exercise program is split up into multiple sections:

► A 10-minute basic program, from page 142
► Exercises for problem areas: back, neck, arms, hips and feet, from page 156
► Tips for Vikings, contortionists and crossover types, from page 191
► Different exercises for men and women, from page 199
► Tips for athletes, from page 210
► Tips for fascia-friendly, creative movements in every day life, from page 221
► Fascia training in older age, from page 225.

This chapter presents descriptions and photographs of the exercises using our two fascia coaches Daniela Meinl and Markus Rossmann as models. All the exercises are drawn from the program of the Fascial Training Academy (see the Appendix for more information and links to the website).

The basic training program consists of six exercises that cover all the important fas-

cial lines. You can start with the basic program and do it twice a week. It takes about ten minutes. You can also integrate it into your existing fitness routine or do a few of the fascia exercises as a warm-up for your usual routine. Feel free to pick and choose other exercises from this chapter according to your personal interests or problems.

In the previous chapters, we have illustrated the importance of considering the body's fascial network as a whole system. This system cannot actually be trained as individual sections or as isolated parts of the body. All of the exercises described here therefore have an impact on the entire system by tapping into the tension network. Conversely, problems, tenseness and matting also radiate out to other parts of the body.

We will still be providing you with exercises and little routines for a few of the known problem areas, such as the back, hips and neck. However, we do recommend that you see these as only one component of your fascia training, rather than as a replacement for the basic program. If you do the basic program twice a week and then build in a few of the following exercises or routines according to your specific needs, you will be giving your fascial network the holistic workout that it needs, and will reap the benefits.

What do you need?

For the training sessions, you will need some simple pieces of equipment, almost all of which are everyday objects: a chair, a tennis ball, small weights, small plastic bottles filled with tap water, and similar objects. Of course, you can also pick up weights, cuff weights, and special rollers and balls from specialist retailers. However, almost all of the exercises can be done perfectly well using everyday objects, so there is really no need to buy new equipment at the beginning.

1. **Filled plastic bottles** Use 500 ml bottles filled with tap water as an alternative to small dumbbells.
2. **Tennis balls** Two standard tennis balls work really well and also make an inexpensive alternative to proper weights.
3. **Stool or footstool** For a few of the exercises, you will need a small, sturdy footstool, which should be about 20 to 30 cm in height. As an alternative, some of the exercises can be done using a step on the stairs.
4. **Balloon** An inflated balloon makes a good cushion for your head.

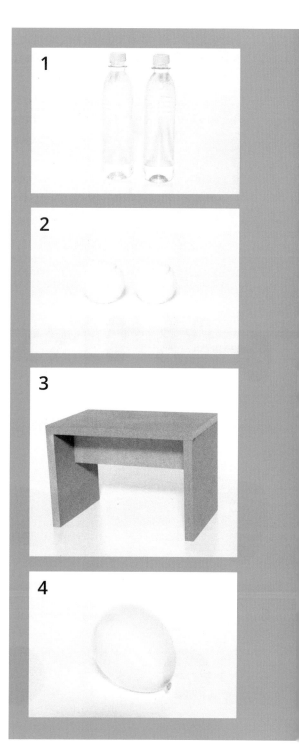

Here is a list of other equipment available from sports shops that you may wish to invest in if you work out regularly:

1. **Small dumbbells** If you already have some, even better! Feel free to increase the weight to 1.5 kg.
2. **Cuff weights** You can get hold of these in various sizes from sports shops. 0.5 to 1 kg per side is plenty.
3. **Nordic walking poles** These poles are great if you need to support yourself with one hand while doing unilateral exercises.
4. **Foam rollers** Rollers come in various degrees of hardness. Blue foam rollers are medium (moderately hard). Black rollers, including the 'BLACKROLL', are hard.

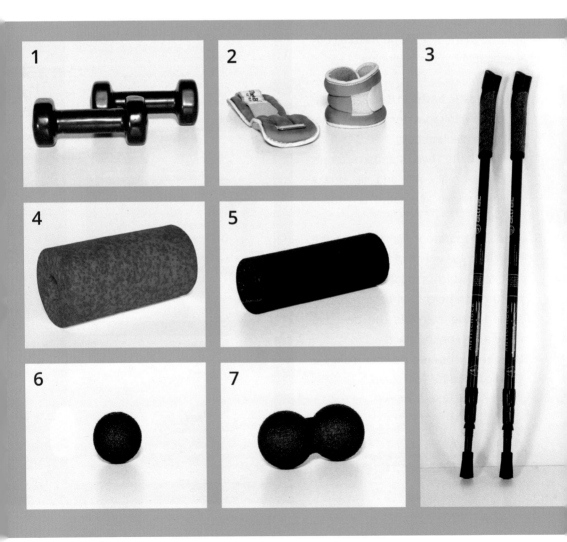

5.–7. Various kinds of fascial roller
There are also various versions of fascia balls or double balls available to buy from specialist shops.

The exception: a special fascia roller

We recommend that you obtain a special foam roller, available from sports shops. It is worth investing in one of these for your fascia training, because it is not an easy thing to substitute with items from around the house. Large filled plastic bottles are usually too soft, balls are too tall and too round, and other training rollers are often too hard for beginners. Simple pool noodles or gymnastics rolls sometimes make a viable alternative, but many people find that these are also too soft. You can buy fascia rollers in specialist shops or on the internet. There is a list of suppliers in the Appendix. These hard foam rollers come in various designs; you may see them referred to by the brand names 'Blueroll' and 'BLACKROLL', or as 'fascia rollers' or 'Pilates rollers'.

You generally have a choice between different degrees of hardness. As a beginner, it is best to start with a medium degree of hardness. Test which roller and which degree of hardness works best for you. For example, you could try an exercise with it in a store, such as rolling out the back of the thighs. To try it out, put some weight on it and see if it feels good. It is fine for it to hurt in a good way ('good pain', as some call it) – like the pleasant pressure you feel when you have a firm massage – but you definitely should not feel a sharp, burning or stabbing pain. You should be able to keep breathing in a relaxed manner. If you notice any sudden twitching in your face or other parts of your body, you find yourself trying to move away from the pressure or it triggers any other protective reactions, then the roller is too hard. So if you find yourself suddenly saying "Ouch!" when testing out the roller, pulling the back of your head down or jerking your shoulders upwards, you should try a softer roller. You will know you have found the right degree of hardness when, after a few breaths, you feel an invigorating dissolving sensation in the tissue.

The rollers usually cost between GBP 20 and 35 (US $27–$45), or at least that is what you would pay for one of the rollers we use in this book. There are cheaper versions available, but we would not recommend them. You will find further information about the different types of roller available in shops – as well as an overview of the possible uses of fascia rollers and balls – in Chapter 4 on pages 250 and 251.

Things to watch out for when using fascia rollers

There are a few safety guidelines to keep in mind when using fascia rollers. You will generally find it beneficial to roll in all directions, as this promotes the exchange of tissue fluid. You may remember the principles behind this from Chapter 2 (pp. 108/109). However, the same does not apply to people who suffer from lymph congestion in their legs. You would be better off rolling from bottom to top, towards the torso, i.e. in the direction of the lymphatic drainage.

Those with weak or varicose veins should also be careful. Before you start using a roller, ask your doctor to show you how to use rollers properly to be on the safe side. In a similar way to compression stockings, which are often prescribed for patients with weak or varicose veins, it is very important to maintain the right level of stimulation when rolling out the fascia on the lower leg. Too little pressure and the exercise may be ineffective; too much and it could be dangerous, so it is definitely worth working out what the right level for you is – as you would with compression stockings – by consulting an experienced specialist.

Clothing and shoes

You can train in regular sports clothes or in yoga attire, or in a T-shirt and sweatpants or leggings. The fabric should be stretchable, comfortable and breathable. You do not need to wear shoes – train with bare feet, including outdoors, as much as you can. This will give you a greater sense of what's happening in your own body.

Many exercises can be done at work or in the office, without having to change. However, you may prefer to choose exercises that don't require you to roll about on the floor when you're at work! Exercises using the foam roller can crease your clothes, so you may wish to choose other exercises for when you're at the office. A thin exercise mat is also useful, but not essential.

Things to consider before you begin

▶ A word of caution to older people and people with underlying illnesses: Fascial exercises are suitable for everyone. However, elderly people or those with long-term conditions such as rheumatism, inflammation or restricted mobility should consult a doctor before commencing the training, as should anyone who has recently undergone surgery or who has an acute injury.

This also applies to those with back pain (where the cause is anatomical), neurological diseases, slipped or herniated discs, or severe osteoporosis, as well as anyone taking blood-thinning medication.

▶ Safety first Make sure you warm up! For all the springing exercises, you must be well warmed up and have a good sense of what's happening in your body, otherwise you could injure yourself. When you plan your own

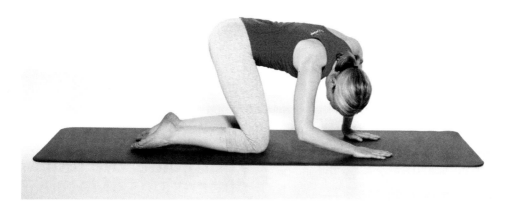

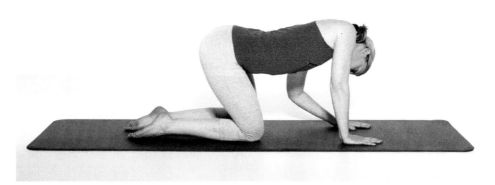

A good exercise for warming up and stimulating the receptors is the 'snake dance', which is described in detail on page 154.

routine using the various exercises, do not start with the springs; begin instead with some warm-up exercises, in particular those from the 'feel' and 'revive' areas. This will activate your receptors and help you to identify your limitations. Warm up well, and gradually increase the intensity.

▶ **Less is more** Try not to over-strain your fascia. Unlike with muscle training, there is no benefit in pushing yourself to the limit of what you can stand. Little and often is best when it comes to your fascia workout – the fascia changes slowly, but the change will last. When you do the 'spring' exercises, it's best to do a few repetitions with breaks in between. When you first start, only do the jumping or swinging exercises three to five times, and then take a short break before you go to the next round. This way, you will allow the tissue time to recover.

▶ **Practice consciously** Always focus when exercising and make sure that your movements feel smooth. Train your perception, do not become distracted when you practice, and do not watch television.

▶ **Practice regularly** You will notice visible signs of improvement after the first training session, but sustainable changes in the structure of your fascia will come after a few months. If you regularly work out twice a week, you will become more supple and flexible. After one year, the entire fascial network in your body will have renewed and reconnected.

▶ **Children should be supervised** Children should not practice on their own, especially not with a foam roller. Fascia training is not suitable for children under six years of age.

▶ **Focus on your breath** Maintaining a good breathing pattern is hugely beneficial in terms of helping you through the exercises and improving how you feel. Have a read through the information about breathing on pages 140 and 141.

Your guide: the four dimensions of fascia training

You will already be familiar with our four training principles from the previous chapter. This circle illustrating the four principles will help guide you through the program: you will find one for every exercise. We will highlight the colour of the area to which the exercise corresponds, which should help you to classify them. If you put a routine together yourself, then you will be able to use the circle to easily find appropriate exercises corresponding to each of the four dimensions. You should always cover all four principles in your individual training program.

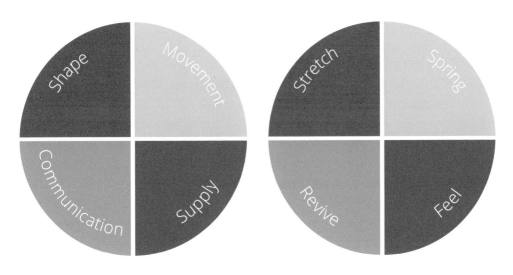

Function: Shape   + Movement   + Communication   + Supply
Training: Stretch   + Spring   + Revive   + Feel

The four training principles correspond to the four basic functions that we learned about in Chapter 2, from page 102. If you concentrate on all four principles of training, you will stimulate the four basic functions of your fascia – and thus provide optimum care and maintenance for your fascial network. The exercises also indicate which of the fascial lines – discussed on pages 72 to 75 – they are designed to activate. You will find the corresponding number on the right, next to the name of each exercise.

If the test clearly showed that you are a contortionist or a Viking, we recommend consulting a doctor or physiotherapist before starting the training. Without advice, you shouldn't go too far down the 'good pain' route with the exercises.

People with weak, easily injured connective tissue should ask a medical professional to show them how to use the fascia roller properly. You can tell if you have weak connective tissue if, for example, you frequently – let's say, several times a year – find that you have a bruise but cannot remember a specific injury. Please also take into consideration the information on the three different types of connective tissue on pages 117 to 119.

Mindful breathing to support your training

When doing the exercises, you will find it useful to know how to use your breath to help you. In everyday life, many people tend to fall into unhealthy breathing patterns. Contrary to popular belief, the problem is not shallow breathing, also known as chest breathing. It is overactive everyday breathing – a sort of intensified air hunger or urge to breathe in more air than the body needs. This excessive inhalation leads to a mild form of biochemical poisoning in the blood, which in turn causes muscles to tense up. It's good to consciously counteract this excessive inhalation in general, but especially so when doing exercises that train fascia, as a supportive breathing pattern will help with your training. In recent years, several studies have shown the benefits of exercises designed to slow the breath, and they can also help us to achieve better results with most of the exercises in this book.

How to use the breath

First things first – put your perfectionist mindset to one side. Direct your attention to what you are feeling in your body at the present moment. Being mindful is about noticing the physical sensations, but also the feelings and emotions that arise or change during the exercise.

Your inhalation should be relaxed and flow naturally. There is no need to set an arbitrary starting point. Try not to actively suck in the air as you breathe. However, you can experiment with opening and stretching movements of the arms or upper body as you inhale. This allows the natural movement when we inhale to reach other parts of the body. In the shoulder exercise on page 170, for example, you can use the stretch to help you breathe into the taut area across your chest as you inhale.

With fast dynamic suspensions, you may wish to make your exhalations more pronounced. In the 'flying sword' exercise on pages 164 and 165, for example, you can breathe out more deeply as you swing your arms downwards. If it doesn't bother your neighbours, try making an audible sound as you exhale. There is an even more powerful version of this, which you can use to activate your pelvic floor. It is described in the instructions for the 'flying sword' exercise on page 165, in the note. For the less dynamic exercises, it is best to simply let the exhalation happen naturally, and observe your breath mindfully and compassionately.

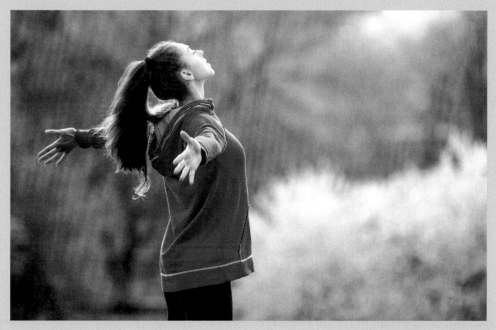

Breathe in deeply and fully during opening movements, as this supports the expansion of fascia.

Soft, gentle exhalations can also support the sensation that we refer to as 'good pain'. This more often occurs during the stretching exercises described in the book or when using a foam roller. So as soon as you feel that familiar sensation of 'good pain' and sense that it is benefiting you, let your breath flow out very slowly and then wait for the inhalation, which will come very gently of its own accord. At first, the inhalation and exhalation movements usually merge seamlessly, with no noticeable pause in between. However, as you become more and more relaxed, you will notice that small pauses naturally occur between the exhale and the next inhale. The more you relax here, the more you will notice that initial feeling of 'good pain' morphing into a pleasant feeling of 'letting go', as the tension melts away.

As studies have shown, after just a few minutes, the gentle exhalation described here begins to calm the autonomic nervous system, which in turn increases overall relaxation and intensifies the regeneration process. Treating fascia with rolling or stretching exercises, combined with this kind of relaxed breathing, can therefore be even more effective at alleviating sleep difficulties and chronic stress than medication.

The basic program

The basic program consists of six exercises and is a daily routine that anyone can do. It is particularly suitable for beginners, those new to sport and those who are a little out of practice. You can influence several important body-wide fascial lines with this compact series of exercises.

Basic training tips

Train for about 10 minutes, once or twice a week. That is plenty for the minimum program. You can of course train more often and longer: three to four times per week is good, depending on your needs. Make sure that exercises from the spring section are performed for the same body part no more than three times a week, and that you allow at least two days' rest between sessions. Exercises from other sections can be performed more often. You should have at least one rest day a week to allow the tissue to recover.

- ▶ A few minutes of repetitions per exercise are plenty – for example, in the morning before work. You can integrate these exercises into your existing fitness regime at home or at work. The basic training program is well-suited to warming up prior to a run or before you play sports.
- ▶ We start with a warm-up and activation, and then move on to foot exercises, followed by back, swinging and neck exercises.
- ▶ Always do the exercises from the basic program in this order to warm up your body, as this will protect against strains and injuries.

The exercises in the basic program

 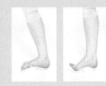

① Rolling out the feet (pp. 144/145)

 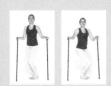

② Elastic jumps for the calves and Achilles tendon (pp. 146/147)

  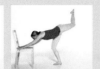

③ Stretching the front and rear lines: eagle flight (pp. 148/149)

④ Stretching the waist and sides: eagle wings on a chair (pp. 150/151)

⑤ Activating the shoulders and shoulder girdle: spring-backs using the arms (pp. 152/153)

⑥ Relaxing the neck and back: snake dance (pp. 154/155).

Rolling out the feet

We start with an exercise from the 'revive' section. Using a tennis ball, roll out the large fascia in the soles of your feet. This is called the plantar fascia. As you perform this, the plantar fascia is filled with new fluid, and different motion and mechanosensors are activated. This exercise is a perfect way to warm up – not just for this program, but for any type of exercise.

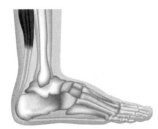

Keeping the foot stable: the plantar fascia.

The plantar fascia runs under the foot from the heel to the ball of the toe, and is one of the thickest sections of fascial tissue in the human body. However, this thick sheet of fascia also needs to be flexible. If not, there can be adverse reactions, such as inflammation or heel spur pain, which can be very painful. Ideally, the heel pad should be able to move forward slightly, which will allow the Achilles tendon to transfer power to the plantar fascia, and the other way around. Rolling your feet over the ball promotes this mobility and boosts metabolism in fascia. This can have positive effects on the back of the leg and also in the hip joints, making them more mobile. They are connected to the plantar fascia via the large dorsal line.

See for yourself Before you start rolling your feet over the tennis ball, bend forward as far as you can on one side with your fingertips pointing towards the floor, but keeping your knee straight. Take a mental note of the distance from your fingertips to the floor. Then do the same thing with the other leg. If you fall into the contortionist category, note the distance from your elbow to the floor. Then do the foot rolling exercise with the leg you tested first. Then bend forward again, with your knee straight and your fingertips pointing towards the floor. Compare the distance with the distance before you did the exercise. I bet you will be amazed at how much more mobile you have become along that whole line!

How it works
1. Stand with bare feet, in a slightly stepped-forward position. Put a tennis ball under the front foot, directly behind the toes.
2. Now, gradually shift more and more weight from the back foot onto the front, and thus onto the ball. Working very slowly, build up until you have as much weight on the

front foot as you can stand. You may find that, in certain spots, you feel a pleasant sort of pain or pressure. This is expected, and indicates the spot where fascia is stuck together. Stay here a moment longer and use small movements to work the ball into this spot.

3. – 5. Then move your foot further forward, rolling the ball away from your toes towards your heel very slowly, as if in slow motion. Try to keep the pressure constant as you go. Let the ball become almost immersed in your foot, and play around with different angles and directions, stimulating the entire sole of the foot. Do this exercise for approximately two minutes, first with one foot, then with the other.

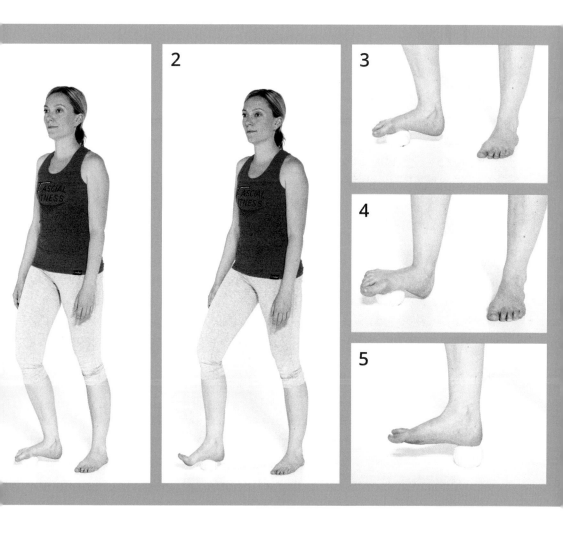

② Elastic jumps for the calves and Achilles tendon

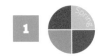

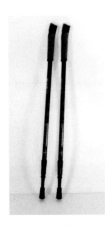

These small, flexible jumps are performed using poles for support, but can also be effective without support. If you want to work with poles, use standard Nordic walking poles.

Elastic jumps specifically train the Achilles tendon, or heel cord. This is the most important tendon for walking and running and has to be tear-resistant and flexible. If the tendon is poorly trained and its supply is inadequate, ensuing problems may lead to Achilles tendon injury. The calf aponeurosis also plays an important role in walking and running. This is an extension of the Achilles tendon, which extends upwards to just below the knee.

Achilles tendon and calf aponeurosis.

Shortening of the Achilles tendon and calf aponeurosis are probably the reason that adults in the Western world often cannot squat down like they did as a child. This is different in other cultures – where squatting to sit down is part of daily life, the tendon remains well-stretched even into adulthood.

We're not saying you'll notice a difference in your tendons overnight, it can take several months to rebuild fascia here. It is therefore well worth practising as often as you can: every time you hop, jump, run barefoot or jog, you encourage the rebuilding of the fascial tissue – but only if you wear special barefoot shoes or no shoes at all. When you first start exercising barefoot, go slowly and carefully, otherwise you will put too much strain on your feet. You can find out more about this on pages 58 to 60.

The elastic jumps below are also a very good exercise for the back, especially the variation described below that includes a twisting movement, because the rotation of the upper body stimulates the fascial sheaths around the intervertebral discs in the spine.

How it works

To prepare yourself, take a few steps in bare feet and apply significant pressure with your heel into the floor. Then begin to push off from the ground a little more quickly with both heels. Be aware of the impact pressure of your heels against the ground.

1. + 2. Then you can start the actual exercise. Rest on the poles and hop slightly upward. When you come back down, try to land as quietly as possible. In other words, try to avoid the foot flopping onto the ground or crashing down onto your heels. The less sound you hear from your feet, the better the exercise!

If you find a sense of ease when you jump, just like a rubber ball, then your fascia is active. Do just three to five repetitions and then take a short break. Keep your heels on the ground or take a few steps on the floor before you start the next round. This is important so that the tissue can recover between the sets of jumps; moreover, through this movement the fluid can be pressed out and then flow back to the fascia again.

Variation

3. + 4. Jump to and fro to the side, or jump in a twisting motion by turning your toes inward and outward. Once you get used to this, you can have a go without the poles. Always make sure to jump as quietly as possible. With time, you will feel that you can consciously control and catch your weight on the toes and front of the foot.

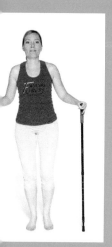
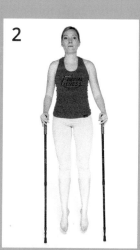
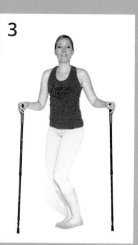
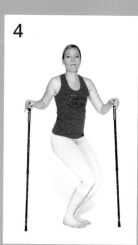

③ Stretching the front and rear lines: eagle flight

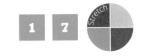

This exercise stretches the connective tissue in the posterior thigh at the hip. It stimulates the long fascial lines in the front and back of the body.

People who spend a lot of time in a seated position often have shortened fascia along the dorsal line and down the legs. You can test this out using the exercise we did earlier before rolling our feet. In a standing position, bend forward, keeping your knees straight. Do your fingertips touch the floor? If not, then the fascia at the rear of your thighs is probably shortened. Because the connective tissue is connected from the thigh up to the sacrum – so, deep into the back – the shortening of this fascial line also affects the lumbar region. This can cause back pain and reduced mobility in the hip joints.

How it works

1. Stand in front of a chair with your feet hip-width apart. Make sure that the chair isn't wobbly. Step back by about a metre and place both hands flat on the seat of the chair. Your weight should be resting mainly on your feet, with your hands placed lightly on the seat.

2. Push your sit bones backward and bend one knee slightly. Push the arm on the same side as far forward as possible. At the same time, stretch the sit bone on the other side as far back as you can.

3. Then switch sides and stretch out the whole of your back side using lolling, spiral-shaped movements and leaning in different directions.

4. To reach the front side, straighten your back and gradually shift your weight forward, bending your elbows. Then slowly lower your upper body towards the seat and give yourself a good stretch. Make sure that you actively draw your lower abdomen inward; otherwise, the weight of the abdominal organs causes the lumbar spine to droop inward and form a hollow in your back. As you do this, actively draw the tips of your shoulder blades down towards your pelvis. Make sure you leave plenty of space between your shoulders and your ears.

5. + 6. Then, roll your back up, keeping your shoulders rounded, slowly returning to the starting position in a big arc.

7. + 8. You can also do other variations of the stretching movements. For example, try arching your back like a cat, then lifting one leg backwards, bending in different positions as you stretch.

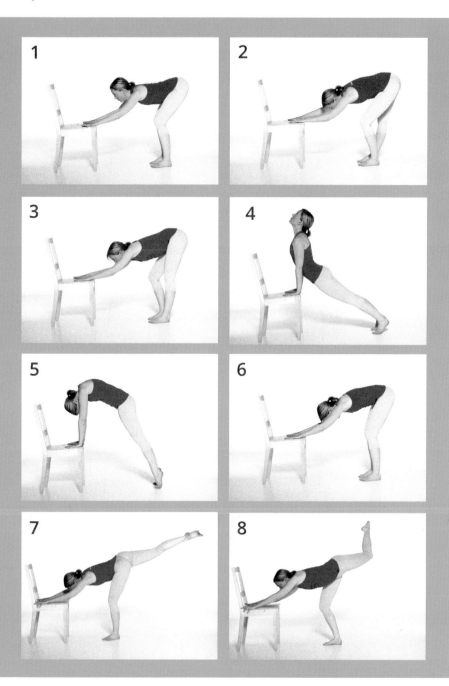

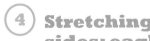 **Stretching the waist and sides: eagle wings on a chair**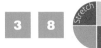

Sitting for long periods, which is an unfortunate aspect of many of our day-to-day lives, results in underuse of the hips, thighs and core. The following exercises are designed to help you stretch out these structures while also stimulating the lateral line that runs through your leg and pelvis, as well as the arm-chest-abdomen line in your upper body. The lateral line and the arm-chest-abdomen line stabilise the core.

How it works

1. Place a stable stool or chair against the wall, making sure it cannot slip. Lean to one side, supporting yourself with one hand on the chair. Both legs should be straight. Extend the whole body as far as possible, making sure that your pelvis does not sag down. The lower side of your body should stay extended throughout.

2. Then, lift your free arm – your upper arm – over your head, tensing that entire side of your body as you stretch it out.

3. + 4. Vary the position of the hand – try stretching your upper arm at different angles and in different directions. Try dipping your arm through the space beneath your body, or reaching it backwards, opening yourself out as far as you can go. You can even experiment with using your own variations.

Note: Make sure that your body is nice and long at all times, and does not sag towards the floor. Keep making little corrections to your posture if you need to. Then, slowly bring yourself back up to a standing position and repeat the exercise on the other side.

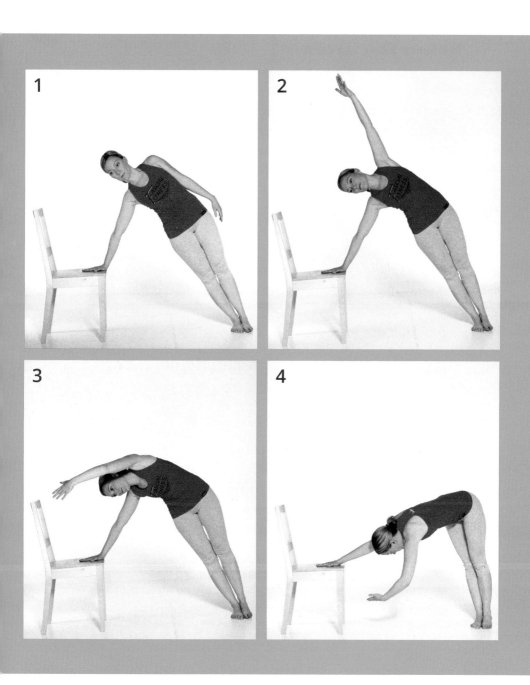

Activating the shoulders and shoulder girdle: spring-backs using the arms

People who spend lots of time sitting at a desk often suffer from shoulder problems. Humans are simply not made to hold that cramped pose for such long periods. The shoulder area contains very firm, thick fascia which connects at the front to the pectoral muscle. The system connects the back and arms at the front of the body, right down to the pelvis. As we evolved, this system is what would have allowed us to swing from tree to tree. Sitting for long periods, especially in an unnatural position such as when working at a desk, leads to tension in many areas of the body.

The fascia in the shoulder joint can become painfully matted, which can lead to shoulder stiffness. In its more extreme manifestation, we refer to this syndrome as 'frozen shoulder'. Keeping our shoulder area flexible and well-trained makes it less prone to stiffness.

The following simple exercise can be carried out on a wall at home or whenever you have a few spare minutes at the office. It is quite versatile, because it trains the abdomen, shoulder and back all at the same time.

How it works
1. + 2. Stand facing the wall, at a distance of between 0.5 and 1 metre. Begin relatively close to the wall, and then increase the distance as you progress. You should be able to tip forward and shift your weight onto your hands. Before you begin, rub your palms together vigorously for a few seconds. This helps to wake up the perceptory sensors in your hands. Then, place your palms flat against the wall and just notice for a moment how your hands feel against the wall. Start by pretending to push the wall away. This activates the structures in the shoulder girdle. Now, push yourself off the wall, letting yourself spring back lightly against the wall. As soon as you make contact with the wall, push off again energetically using both hands.

Variation
3. + 4. Repeat the exercises six or seven times. Then you can try the variations. Place your hands diagonally to the left, then to the right, and so on.

Note

▶ Notice how the movement works a bit like a rubber ball: springing back against the wall should feel easy and effortless, as if it were a trampoline. If it feels really strenuous, as if you were doing a press-up against the wall, then you are working too much with your muscles and not enough with your fascia. In this case, move closer to the wall and try to use the springiness of your fascia to find a dynamic, effortless rhythm.

▶ Pull the lower abdomen slightly inward to stabilise your core and also to avoid a hollow back.

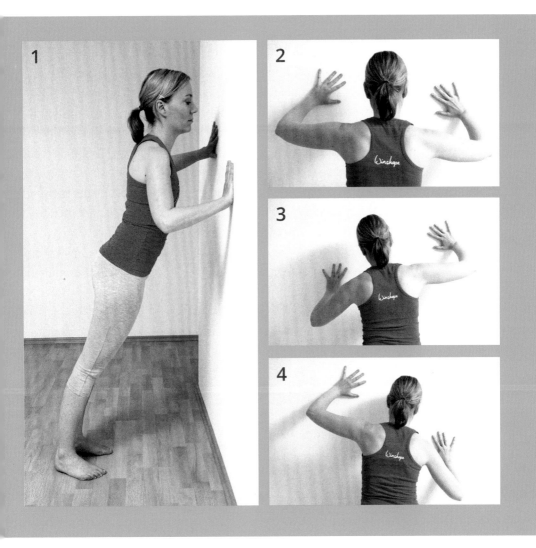

⑥ Relaxing the neck and back: snake dance

Neck pain frequently occurs in combination with a headache. That is no coincidence: the neck fascia runs from the back of the head, up and over the head, all the way to the eyebrows. A little further down the neck, around the shoulders, the fascia is very soft. The neck has to be very flexible so that you have sufficient mobility to turn your head easily. When it comes to the fascia in your neck, it is therefore important to do exercises that firm it, while also retaining its flexibility. In all the exercises around the neck, you should proceed very gently and slowly.

How it works

1. Position yourself on all fours, knees bent, on the floor or on a mat. Your knees should be hip-width apart and your arms should be in line with your shoulders.

2. Using slow, snake-like movements, start to move through your spine, making it undulate like a wave. Lift your sternum, round your back and then let your sternum sink down towards the floor. Keep the lumbar spine still and stretch the tailbone. The movement should be fluid and feel quite pleasant.

3. – 5. Now try some lateral oscillations: move in larger sideways movements between the shoulders, back and forth, then finally in a figure of eight and in a circular motion.

6. – 8. Experiment with different directions, angles and wave movements. The whole exercise should last a few minutes. As you come to the end of the exercise, make your movements smaller and more delicate, gradually coming to a stop. Spend a moment just noticing how your body feels.

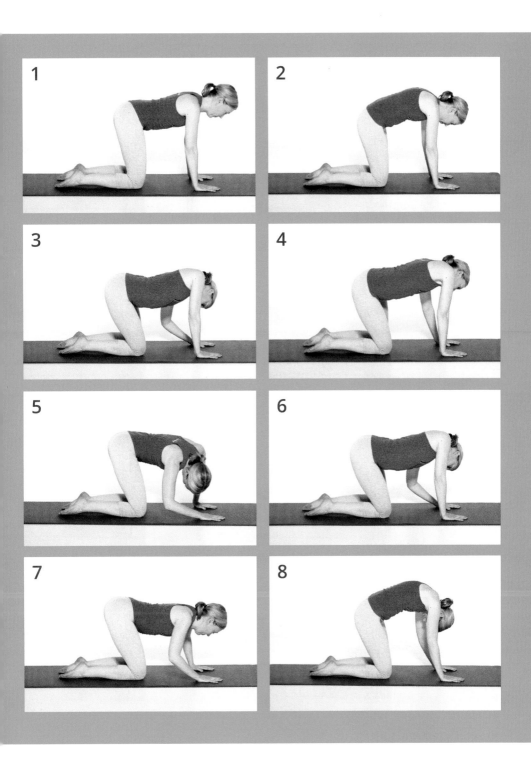

Exercises for problem areas: back, neck, arms, hips and feet

The following series of exercises cover the individual problem areas or issues from various different angles. Always think of fascia as a whole network, and try to train in a way that works for your whole body. You can do this by integrating the short series of exercises, or particular exercises of your choosing, into your regular basic training.

Programs for problem areas
► A short program for back problems (pp. 157–167)
► Office pains: problems in the neck, arms and shoulders (pp. 168–175)
► The hip area (pp. 176–182)
► For the feet and gait (pp. 183–190).

A short program for back problems

Here is a mini workout for the back – five exercises, specifically aimed at the lumbar fascia, and covering all four training dimensions. It specifically protects against back pain but is also good for anyone who spends long periods standing or sitting in one position.

You can do these exercises two or three times a week, or add them to your usual workout. At least for the first few times, it is recommended to follow this order.

An overview of the exercises

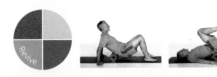

① Rolling out the lumbar fascia
(pp. 158/159)

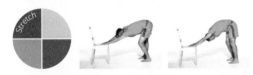

② Stretching the back: the cat
(pp. 160/161)

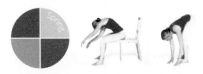

③ African bends
(pp. 162/163)

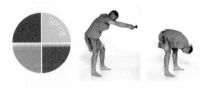

④ Flying sword
(pp. 164/165)

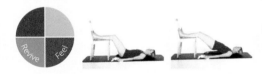

⑤ Relieving the spinal chain
(pp. 166/167)

This little series of exercises makes up one basic program. According to recent findings, exercises that involve rotating the spine are especially good for the back (see page 53 on the topic of back pain). So, if you really want to do your back a favour and find relief from back pain, we recommend that you add the following three exercises onto exercise 4, the 'flying sword', and then do the 'relieving the spinal chain' exercise to finish off the routine:

- ► The flamingo (pp. 205/206)
- ► Throwing (page 207)
- ► Elastic springs with twisting movements (page 189).

① **Rolling out the lumbar fascia**

We start with rolling out the lumbar fascia, which stimulates the tissue and promotes fluid exchange, so that fascia can regenerate and repair damage. This is where the fascia roller comes into play. If you want to do back exercises more often, then a fascia roller is really worthwhile; we also work with a fascia roller for thigh and calf exercises.

How it works

1. Sit comfortably on the floor or on a mat and place your hands on the floor behind you to prop yourself up. Then lift up your pelvis and place the fascia roller crossways underneath your lumbar region.

2. Roll upwards a little toward the chest and then back again, keeping your arms crossed behind your head.

3. Next, stretch out your arms to open up your shoulder girdle. Roll slowly up and down.

4. Now lift your legs in the air, keeping the fascia roller underneath your lower back. Do this consciously and slowly. Spread your hands to the sides on the floor. Try to keep your back nice and round and make sure the roller is not in the hollow of your back.

5. + 6. Now, very slowly as if in slow motion, start to vary your position on the roller in small angles. Keep changing the position of the fascia roller until you have rolled out your entire back fascia.

Note

▸ Try to control the pressure, so that the experience feels like a back massage. You should not feel any acute or sharp sensations.

▸ If lying down is difficult, you can do the exercise standing up against a wall, with support from your legs. You might be able to control the pressure more easily in this position.

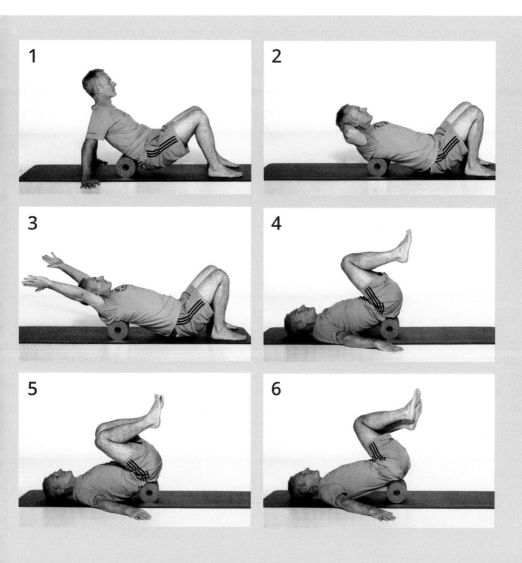

② Stretching the back: cat

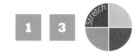

How it works

1. Take a chair and place it with the backrest against a wall. Step back by about a metre and place both hands flat on the seat of the chair. If you don't have a chair, use the windowsill. Your weight rests mainly on your feet, with the hands placed lightly on the seat.

2. Stand with your feet about hip-width apart, with your arms extended and your hip joints positioned above the heels. Bend your knees slowly forward and simultaneously press your tailbone back and up like a cat, extending while stretching your buttocks upward.

Now let the right sit bone come back up, extending your right knee and shifting your weight onto your left foot. Spread the fingers of your right hand and slide them forward onto the seat of the chair. You should feel a deep stretch down your right side. Relax for a moment, and then repeat the exercise with the left side.

3. Keeping your back rounded right down to your coccyx will mostly reach the superficial layer of the lumbar fascia. So, once you have done the first round of stretches, try repeating the exercise, keeping your back straight. This will allow you to reach the deeper layer as well. Make sure to actively draw your lower abdomen inward; otherwise, the weight of your abdominal organs will cause the lumbar spine to droop inward and create a hollow in your back. Can you feel a pull down the back of your legs? Excellent! That means you're doing it right.

Variation: If you like a bit more of a challenge, then you can try this exercise while standing up without the chair.

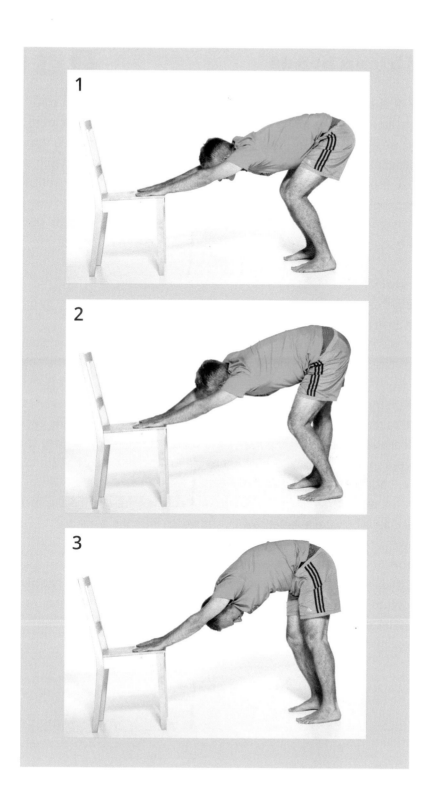

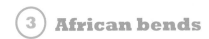 **African bends**

Not only does the back fascia distribute load and hold the muscles in place – it also appears to act like a huge spring when we walk. That is why, if we are trying to address back pain, we also want to increase the elastic storage capacity of the lumbar fascia – by activating those springs deep in the back. This bending exercise is based on movements that researchers have observed in some regions of Africa. While working on the fields, the people there do similar suspensions with their backs. Although they are bent over, this is a remarkably natural and gentle posture that capitalises on the storage power of fascia.

How it works
1. Sit upright on the front edge of a stable chair and open your legs slightly more than hip width apart.
2. Lower your chin onto your chest and slowly roll your spine forwards and down, until your fingertips touch the ground. Your knees should stay in line with the tips of your toes.
3. + 4. Now try to pull yourself a tiny bit further down toward the floor. This will cause the fascia to tense slightly. Now let go and your lumbar fascia will spring back. Find a rhythm that suits you, so that the movement does not put you under any strain. You should feel a springy feeling, as though there is a rubber ball bouncing up and down in your lower back.
5. – 7. Again, play with small changes in the angle of the arms and the alignment of the lower back, as if you were energetically pulling weeds from the ground.

Variation
8. – 11. If you feel confident, you can do this exercise while standing. Try it bent about halfway over to begin with, and then try bending all the way to the ground. Your knees should not be locked, but slightly bent.

Note: Some people can naturally keep their backs straight when doing these sorts of exercises **(9)**, while others find their spine is naturally more rounded **(11)**. This largely depends on how flexible you are. However, the main thing to focus on here is to activate that elastic, springing movement – not to keep a straight back.

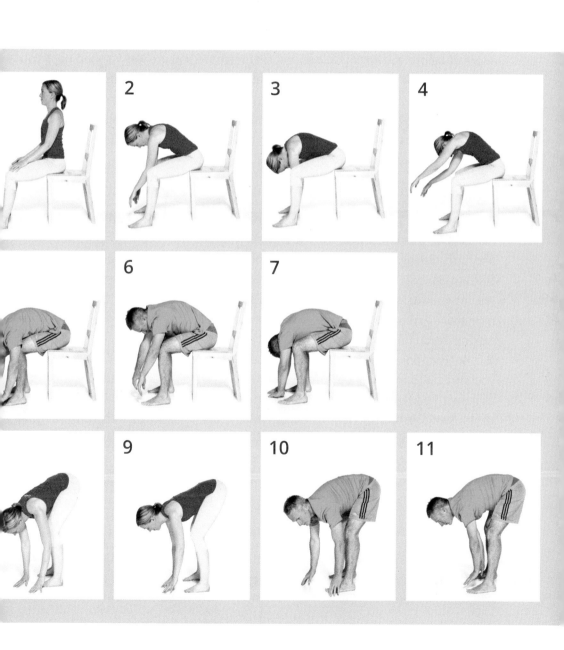

(4) Flying sword

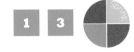

This exercise not only targets the lumbar fascia, it also incorporates the large dorsal line, as well as the line that runs between the arm, chest and abdomen. They are particularly important for our core strength and stability.

The 'flying sword' is very intense and energetic, so there are a couple of things to be aware of before you begin: Only do the exercise once you are well warmed up. If you suffer from back pain or any sort of spinal instability, such as a slipped disc, take it easy at the start. First try one or two gentle repetitions, so that you can detect whether this exercise has a stabilising or destabilising effect on your lower back, which depends largely on your personal body structure. In the case of the latter, or if you are unsure, do not do this exercise.

How it works

1. Hold a small 1.5 kg dumbbell (or, alternatively, a small, filled water bottle) in both hands. Raise the dumbbell up over your head. Now, start to move your upper body back and forth, making slow, snake-like movements. This pre-loads the fascia in the torso and starts to generate the momentum that you will need for the next movement. The snake-like movements should pass through the stomach and chest, and there should be movement of the thoracic spine. Do five or six repetitions of these movements while holding the dumbbell behind your head.

2. – 4. Now spring forward from your sternum. Bring your upper body down and swing your arms with the dumbbell passing backward between your legs and then back up over your head. Straighten your arms naturally into the swing. Do this smoothly and gently. Swing six or seven times, from top to bottom and back again. Then, try swinging to the left and right sides on your way back up. Repeat this a total of at least 20 times. When swinging backwards with your arms stretched above your head, make sure that there isn't too much of a hollow in your lower back; otherwise you can strain the area.

Note

▶ If you notice during this exercise that you tend to overstretch your lower back when your stomach is relaxed, then try to keep your lower abdomen and waist pulled in slightly as you stretch.

- On the down-swing, try making an audible sound as you exhale. This will help to support your breathing.
- There is a particularly intense variation of this, whereby you can activate your pelvic floor by imagining that the sound is coming from your lower abdomen and pelvic area.

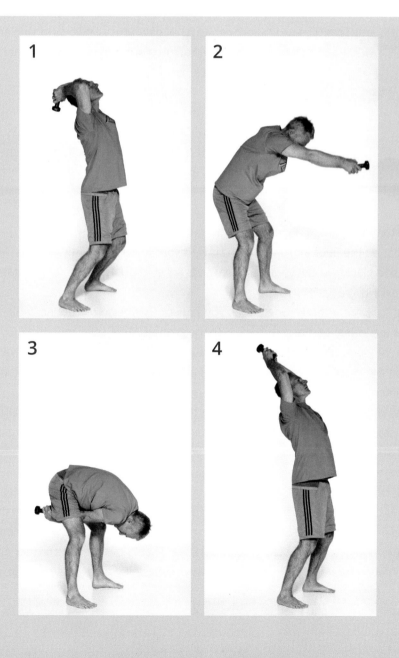

⑤ Relieving the spinal chain

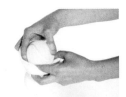

The spinal column is not like a column at all, but instead resembles a flexible chain. As you learned in Chapter 2, what keeps it stable and upright is the system of fascial tension. We therefore refer to the backbone as the 'spinal chain' in this exercise, the primary aim of which is to restore its flexibility. We will do this in a wide variety of ways, all of which will help to loosen and rejuvenate the fascial structures around the muscles that hold the spinal chain in place.

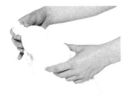

For this exercise, you will need two tennis balls wrapped in a sock or stocking. Tie a knot above the tennis balls to stop them flying out. Alternatively, a double ball which is specifically designed for such exercises can be purchased from a sports shop.

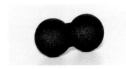

How it works

1. Lie flat on the floor in front of a chair, with your lower legs resting on the seat. You can place a blanket under your pelvis or calves for comfort. Hold the sock containing the tennis balls in your hand.

2. First, loosen the back generally as you consciously begin to connect your sacrum, which is the lowest part of your back, with the ground. Make small tentative movements toward the floor with the lower part of your back. Then, slowly lift your whole spinal chain off the ground and move one vertebra at a time back to the ground. Repeat this three times.

3. Now, lift up your lower back and push the sock containing the tennis balls under your thoracic spine, so that the balls are placed either side of the spine. The gap in the middle should leave plenty of space for your spinous processes to sit comfortably between the two balls. Only continue if you feel that the balls are contacting muscle and not bone.

4. – 6. Now, slowly bring your weight down onto the balls, gradually increasing the pressure. Again, you can make small angle changes to the contact points with the balls. Stay in this position as long as you find it comfortable. Then move the balls further down the back, one vertebra at a time, and repeat the exercise. By doing this exercise, you will work down to the sacrum step by step. At this point, remove the balls and just feel how your back feels against the floor for a moment. Do you notice a change?

Note: The twisting versions of the flamingo, throwing and elastic jumps exercises are ideal for this.

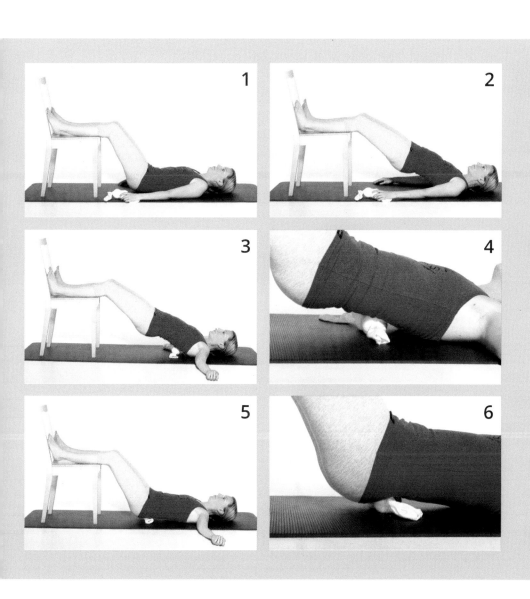

Office pains: problems in the neck, arms and shoulders

The fascia of the spinal and lateral lines is not utilised efficiently when sitting continuously. When working at a desk, or looking at a computer screen, your arms usually rest in an unfavourable position on the desk. Syndromes affecting the shoulders, neck and arms are common issues arising from sitting for long periods, even more so than deep lower back pain. The following short series of exercises relieves the strained fascia in this area and stimulates the long fascial lines that connect the arms, torso and legs with one another, but deteriorate when sitting for long periods.

These exercises can be done at home or at the office, or you can use them twice a week to enhance your regular fascia program. The swinging exercise 'swinging bamboo' on pages 174 and 175 should only be done after the body has been warmed up or at the end of the series of exercises. The shoulder exercise 'spring-backs using the arms' from the basic program on pages 152 and 153 can also be integrated into this series – ideally at the end.

An overview of the exercises

 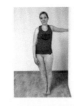

① Stretching the shoulders (page 170)

② Freeing up the neck (page 171)

 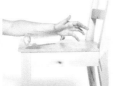

③ Relaxation for tired forearms (pp. 172/173)

 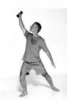

④ Momentum for the whole body: swinging bamboo (pp. 174/175).

Stretching the shoulders

How it works

1. Stand in the door frame or by a wall or cabinet, as shown in the image. Place your hand flat on the surface, then move a little forward and stretch the arm and shoulder.

2. + 3. You can experiment with small angle changes to activate the different fibres. Change the position of your hand too – sometimes higher, sometimes lower. Change the angle of your body to the wall as well to vary the stretch.

Note: Try to notice where the stretch feels particularly good for you. Experiment with this.

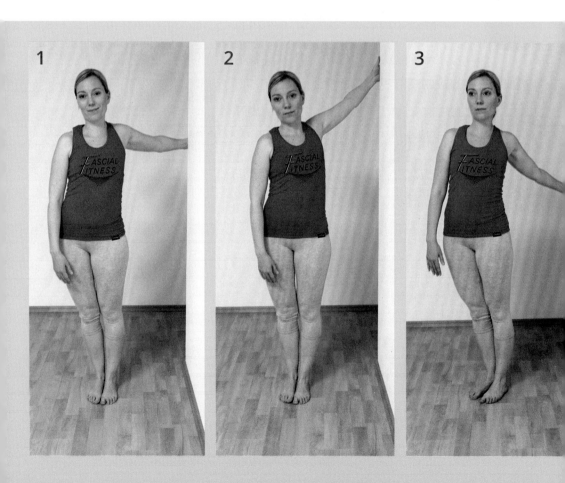

② Freeing up the neck

This exercise relieves the cervical spine and all the fascial elements around the neck, shoulders and head. Only rarely do we sit so precisely aligned that the weight of the head rests just above the spinal chain, which would be the ideal posture. As a result, the muscles need to do a lot of balancing work, which can cause the entire shoulder area to become tense and the cervical spine to be overloaded. With this exercise, you can loosen this particular area of your neck.

How it works

1. You will need an inflated balloon for this exercise. Position yourself in front of a chair, with your legs hip-width apart, and hold the balloon in your hand. Tighten your abdomen a little and roll, vertebra by vertebra, down to the seat of the chair. Place the balloon on the seat and put the top of your head on the balloon. Place your hands loosely on the seat to support you.

Experiment with small angle changes in the neck: try touching the balloon to the crown of your head, and rolling it gently back and forth. Control the weight of your head on the balloon – do not press too hard. Your neck should stay loose and relaxed. Try to make your movements gradually smaller and more varied.

2. It is even more challenging if you do this exercise without a balloon, and just with your head placed directly on the seat of the chair.

Variation: As you become more advanced, try practising the exercise on the floor, on all fours, with or without a balloon.

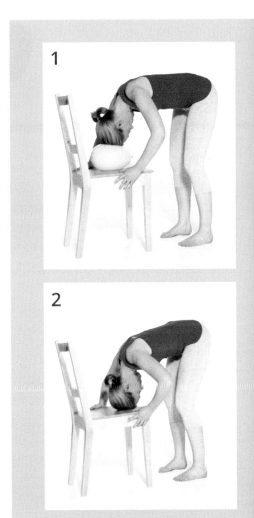

③ **Relaxation for tired forearms**

This exercise is ideal for when you have a few spare minutes in your work day, especially when your forearms are suffering from being in the same position for too long. You will need a small, filled water bottle or a small fascia roller (see image: mini roller by BLACKROLL, 15 cm long, 5.4 cm thick).

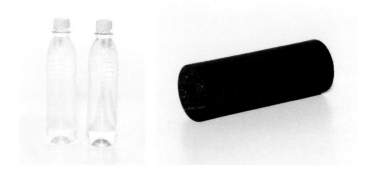

How it works

1. Place the water bottle or roller in front of you on the table, desk or chair. Rest your forearm on top.

2. + 3. Now, put as much weight on the bottle or roller so that it is just at the edge of your comfort zone. Then, start to slowly roll out your forearm, millimetre by millimetre. Roll lengthways from elbow to hand or the other way round. As you roll, play around with lots of little angle changes.

Note: Do this really, really slowly and try to imagine that you are pressing out water from a sponge. The pressure of the bottle or roller creates little ripples in the fascia. Slowly push these out.

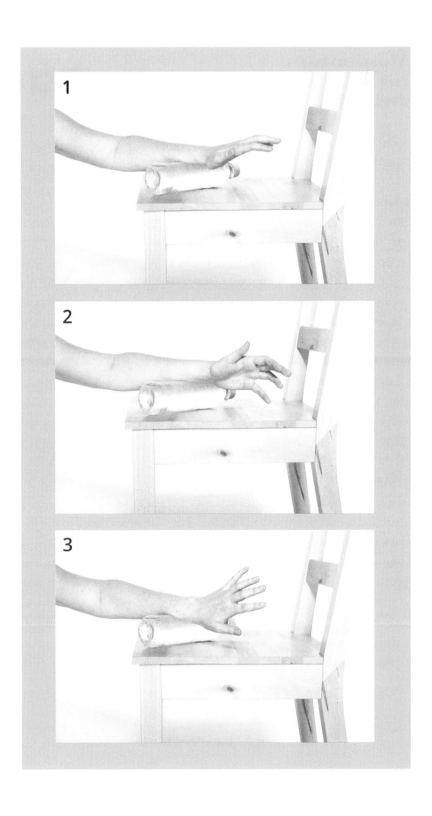

④ Momentum for the whole body: swinging bamboo

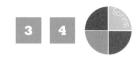

For this exercise you will need a small dumbbell, about 0.5 to 1.5 kg in weight. Alternatively, you can use a small filled water bottle.

How it works

1. + 2. Stand in a stable position, a bit like a sumo wrestler. We call this pose the 'stand of strength'. Your legs should be slightly further than hip-width apart, with the tips of your toes pointing outwards slightly. Your knees should be slightly bent, so that they extend just beyond the tips of your toes. Make sure that your back is straight and there is not a pronounced curve in the small of your back. Imagine a small weight pulling your tailbone down. Holding the dumbbell with both hands in front of your body, start by swinging it in small circles around the spinal chain. This will gradually warm up the fascia. Perform these circle swings for about a minute.

3. Then, swing diagonally up and back to one side for a few repetitions, before adding in your legs. To do this, bend your knee on the side you are swinging towards, straightening your other leg. Try opening your arms as you swing. When you swing to the right, release your grip on the dumbbell (or bottle) with your left hand. Swing with your right arm, with the dumbbell in your hand, diagonally upward to the right, and rotate the torso up to the right. This creates tension in the fascial lines at the front of your body – in this instance, the diagonal torso line and the arm-chest-abdomen line.

Make sure that the outer edge of your left foot stays firmly anchored to the floor. When you do the exercise on the other side, do the same with your right foot.

4. + 5. Remain in this position for a moment. Here, do little bounces to intensify the stretch from the outer edge of your foot, up through the straightened leg, all the way to the hand that is holding the dumbbell. Now use the momentum from the bounce to spring back down again: stretch your whole side like an arch and swing diagonally back down, leading with the chest area. Try to make the movement follow a smooth curve and do not overstretch yourself!

Note: Listen to your body! Once you feel that you have understood the physics of the movement, then you can perform three to five repetitions in the upper position without a break. Relax, then switch to the other side.

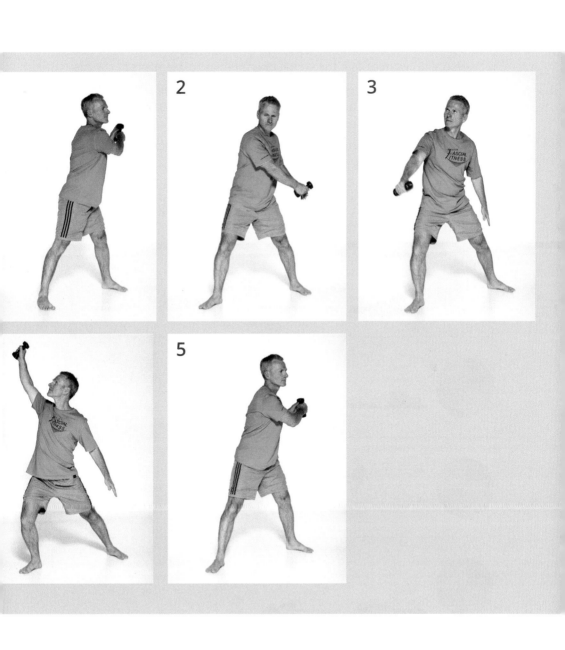

The hip area

Because pain and loss of motion at the hip joint are very common, this small set of exercises for the hips will appeal to many people. Hip surgery is unfortunately one of the most frequent operations in the Western world. After the knee, the hip is the next largest joint in the human body; it contains the strongest ligaments of the entire body. It is therefore no wonder that the condition of the fascial elements in the hip has such a major impact on our mobility. In each step we take, the hip joints and ligaments are used, and this joint must be extremely mobile. However, regularly sitting for long periods at a time results in unhelpful lengthening of one side of the hip, while also underutilising the joint. This also restricts the supply of nutrients to the cartilage in the joint. Certain sports, such as cycling, are also not ideal for the supply and mobility of the hip, and we should therefore compensate for this with appropriate exercises.

An overview of the exercises

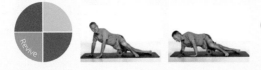 ① Rolling out the outer thighs (page 177)

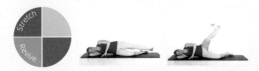 ② Activating the outer thighs (pp. 178/179)

 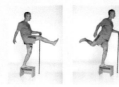 ③ Swinging the legs (pp. 180/181)

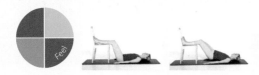 ④ The skate (page 182).

① **Rolling out the outer thighs**

You will need a fascia roller for this exercise.

How it works

1. Assume the starting position by lying on your right side, with your weight on the right hand, so that your elbow is below the right armpit. Place the foam roller just below the femoral head of your right leg, i.e. the rounded bony protruberance at the top of your thigh (the trochanter). Now straighten out the bottom leg and pull the top leg up and over the right leg. Use your free hand – your left hand – to support your upper body.

2. Now, slowly roll down from the trochanter, down the outer side of your thigh, toward the knee. As you press slowly over the roller, imagine your thigh is a sponge. If you find areas that are particularly tight or painful, hold the position for half a minute to a minute, and relax slowly into the pressure while making tiny angle changes. Make sure to keep your head in line with your spine. You can also do the exercise with your right arm bent and the forearm supported on the ground, taking the weight of the upper body.

When the roller reaches a point just above the knee, slowly roll back up to the trochanter. After the second pass, you may already feel a soothing 'dissolving' sensation in the tissue. Finally, remove the roller and feel the release in your thigh.

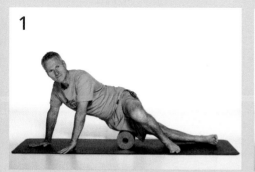

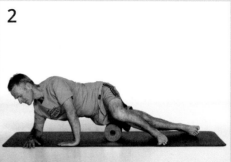

② **Activating the outer thighs**

How it works

1. Lie down on your side on the floor. Your bottom leg should be slightly bent, with the upper leg floating in a slightly raised position above the ground. Be sure to stretch your back and to not allow your spine to sag sideways (down).

2. Next, bend the knee of the top leg and slide your foot out from the leg in front of the body, as if you wanted to push a wall away.

3. When you reach full knee extension, stretch a bit further out at the heel and then through each individual toe. Make sure that you stay in the side position. Bend your knee slightly and slide your leg out again like a telescope, this time by extending the lumbar chain down and out.

4 + 5. Adjust the motion by making small rotational changes and using various angles; slide the leg in different directions – upward, forward and diagonally. To change sides, slowly curl up with your knees drawn to your chest and roll over onto the other side.

Variation

6. + 7. If you are looking for a bigger challenge, instead of lying down on the ground you can position yourself sideways on a chair, or you could put on cuff weights. However, always make sure that you have enough stability in the trunk and cervical chain, so as not to overload these structures.

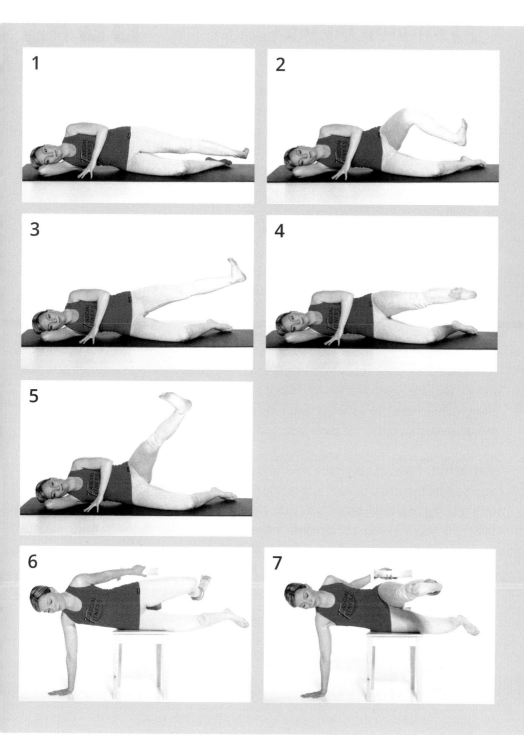

③ Swinging the legs

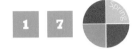

How it works

1. This exercise is best done with bare feet. Stand on a low stool and use one of your Nordic walking poles for support. Start on the left side and lean your weight onto the pole with your left hand, keeping the right hand free. Your left foot should be planted securely on the stool, with the knee slightly bent, and your right foot should be hanging loosely by your side. Now begin to swing your right leg loosely back and forth. Keep the movement slow, so that your leg swings forwards and backwards like a pendulum.

2. – 4. Now, let's concentrate on the fascial momentum. Move your free leg back carefully and stretch the tissue backward, letting your leg spring forward out of your pelvis. Try not to be tempted to use the muscle to bring the left forward and upwards. Instead, make sure that you are using the momentum in the fascia itself, which should be pre-loaded with the energy it stored during the back-swing. Then, the spring mechanism of the fascia comes into play.

Swing the entire leg back and forth smoothly in a rhythmic motion. Feel your hip and the whole side of the upper body to the right, and in front over the chest to the left arm. You can increase the catapult effect by making sure that the momentum that drives the leg swing comes from the tension created by pulling back your pubic bone. After about three minutes, switch to the other side.

Variation: Once you are more advanced, try the exercise without the pole. You can also do it on the stairs, or even just on the floor, after a little practice. To do this, stand with your legs hip-width apart, shift your weight to one leg and swing the other. In the beginning, you may wish to hold onto a windowsill or chair with one hand to maintain your balance. This will help you focus on swinging your free leg. However, once you feel more confident with the exercise, try doing it without the support.

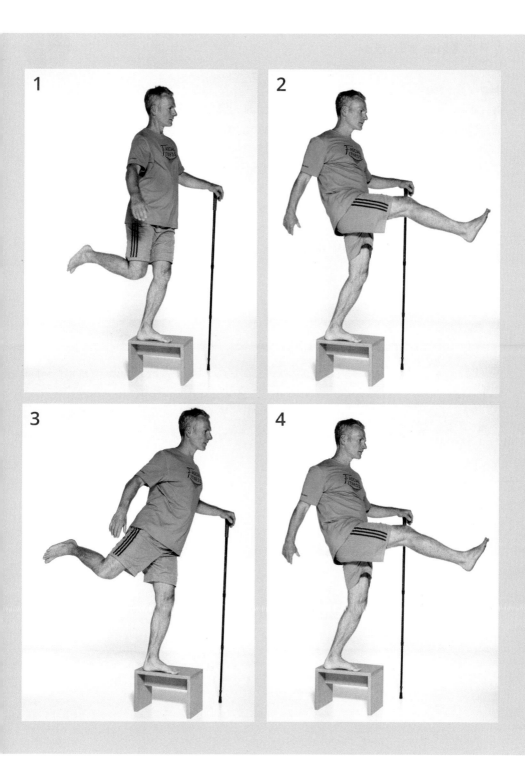

④ **The skate**

How it works

1. Lie flat on your back in front of a stable chair and place your lower legs onto the seat in a parallel position. Start by placing your sacrum (the lowest part of your pelvis) on the floor. Try different contact points and touching it to the floor at different angles.

2. Next, slowly lift up your pelvis by extending your tailbone. Now use different curves, spirals and waves with your raised pelvis – like a skate meandering through the sea. Proceed slowly and deliberately, and be aware of your inner impulses for the next move. Finally, let your pelvis sink gently down to the floor, vertebra by vertebra, before launching into the next round. Repeat three times.

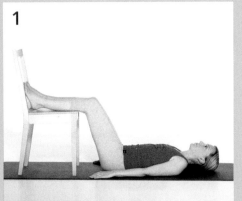

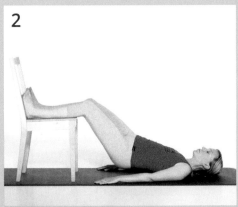

For the feet and gait

Thanks to the catapult effect of the muscles and tendons, walking is the most energy-efficient mode of transport for people. How well this works depends on the body's awareness and balance, and on the elastic storage capability of fascia. Another significant element of our walking ability are the long fascial lines that we saw in Chapter 2: the diagonal torso line or spiral line. The diagonal torso line is responsible for balance and tracking when walking.

The following short series of exercises shows you how to practice several important functions relating to the feet and posture. People who walk a lot, and also those who spend a significant amount of time standing, should regularly stretch their Achilles tendon. Others who spend lengthy periods on their feet can create a lot of energy by regularly strengthening the fascia in the feet and lower legs with elastic jumping. We begin and end this series with exercises for vitality and awareness.

An overview of the exercises

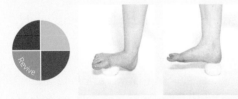

① Rolling out the plantar fascia (page 185)

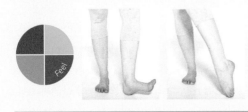

② Sensitising the soles of the feet (pp. 186/187)

  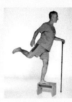

③ Swinging the legs (page 188)

 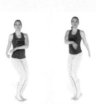

④ Elastic jumps for the feet, calves and Achilles tendon (page 189)

 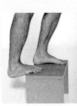 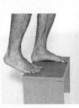

⑤ Stretching the Achilles tendon (page 190)

Rolling out the plantar fascia

For this exercise you will need a tennis ball. Begin by rolling out the plantar fascia as in exercise 1 of the basic program, described in detail on pages 144 and 145. Put particular emphasis on the heel pad.

How it works

1. Stand with bare feet, in a slightly stepped-forward position. Put a tennis ball under the front foot, directly behind the toes. Now gradually shift more and more weight from the back foot onto the front, and thus onto the ball of the foot. Working very slowly, build up until you have as much weight on the front foot as you can stand. You may find that, in certain spots, you feel a pleasant sort of pain or pressure. This is expected, and indicates the spot where the fascia is stuck together. Stay here a moment longer and use small movements to work the ball into this spot.

2. Then move your foot further forward, rolling the ball away from your toes towards your heel very slowly, as if in slow motion. Try to keep the pressure constant as you go. Let the ball become almost immersed in your foot, and play around with different angles and directions, stimulating the entire sole of the foot. Do this exercise for approximately two minutes, first with one foot, then with the other.

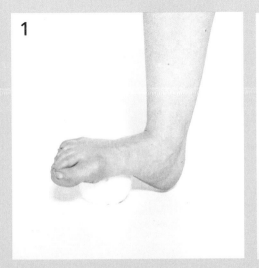

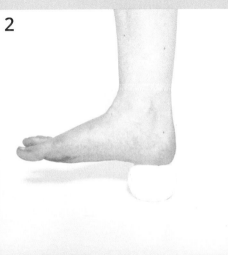

(2) Sensitising the soles of the feet

How it works

1. – 6. Stand with your legs hip-width apart. Shift your weight to one side and begin to touch the floor with the sole of your free foot in a very conscious way, making tiny micro-movements. Play with different amounts of pressure, pushing different bits of the foot into the ground and noticing how it feels. Proceed slowly and work your way over the entire sole of the foot. Next, take a moment to relax on both legs. Have you noticed the difference? The exercise can even have a relaxing effect on the entire body. Repeat the exercise on the other side.

Variation

7. Try this exercise on different surfaces – carpet, tile, wood or a mat – or with a towel under your foot. Consciously note the differences.

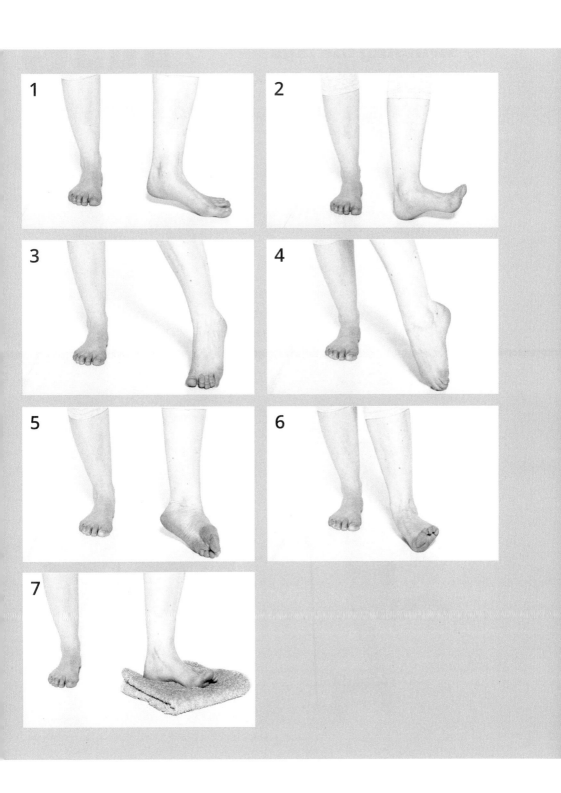

③ Swinging the legs

How it works

This exercise has already been described in the series of exercises for the hips on pages 180 and 181. The hip movement that you practice can even be used while walking. This is what's known as the 'pendulum walk', which is particularly energy efficient as long as you stay in your own rhythm. This is something you will probably have noticed if you go hiking or take a walk with other people. If you try to go too fast or walk at someone else's pace instead of your own, it takes up a lot more energy. In short, we tend not to walk in the optimum way for our bodies. Or as we fascia researchers would say, we don't tap into the power of our fascia!

Have a go at this little walking meditation next time you're out and about: pre-load your back leg **(1)** as you learned in the swinging exercise; then relax it just as you take your next step forward **(2)**. This should make it spring forwards by itself. Try to find your own rhythm. With this exercise, you will improve the use of your fascia and save muscle energy.

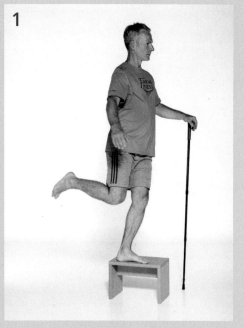

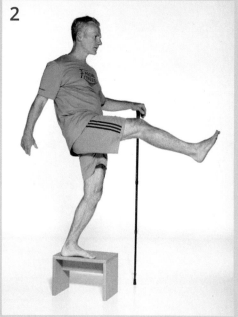

Elastic jumps for the feet, calves and Achilles tendon

How it works

You should also be familiar with this exercise by now, too. It is the elastic jumps from the basic program on pages 146 and 147. These jumps specifically train the Achilles tendon and all the muscles and fascia in the feet and lower legs. This exercise can be performed with or without poles, and is best done barefoot.

1. + 2. Jump to and fro to the side, or jump in a twisting motion by turning your toes inward and outward. Always try to land as quietly as possible. With time, you will feel that you can consciously control and catch your weight on the toes and front of the foot.

Note: As we have already discussed, to maintain a smooth and energy-efficient gait, you need to include a variety of different movements in your day-to-day life, be it hopping, jumping, running barefoot or dancing.

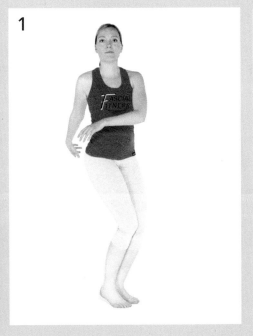

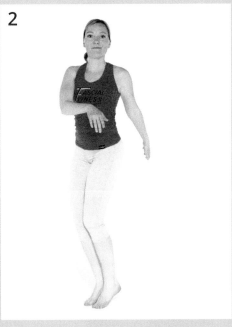

⑤ Stretching the Achilles tendon

We have already seen how important the condition of the Achilles tendon is from the exercises for the basic program (page 142). Stretching the Achilles tendon is particularly important for those who run regularly and spend long periods standing up – but even more so for older people, for Viking types with stiff tissues, and for athletes.

How it works

1. Stand on a stool. Pull back one heel a little and let it float freely, while keeping the other foot flat on the stool.

2. + 3. Now push the floating heel down and hold this position for a few moments. Then vary the position of the heel using small angle changes to achieve a stretch in the various fibres.

Note: Take care not to overstretch, and decide when you need to rest for a while. Maintain the whole body erect and tense. You can also stretch your arms up above your head in order to involve the whole body. Instead of a stool, you could use a step on the stairs for this exercise.

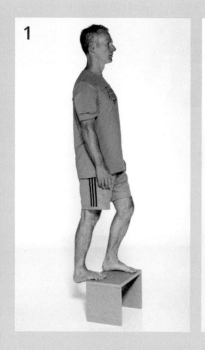

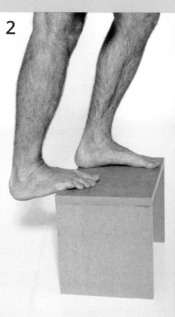

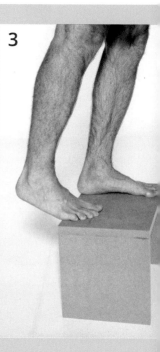

For Vikings, contortionists and crossover types

Tips and exercises

This section presents some important information and exercises that are particularly useful for the various types of connective tissue, especially the ones at either end of the scale.

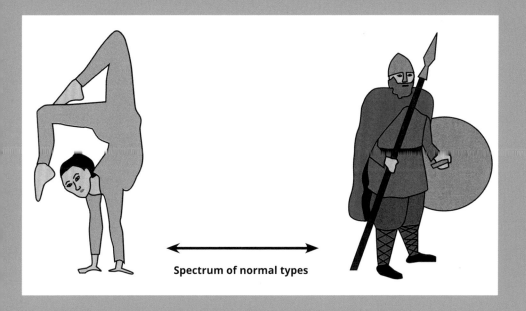

Spectrum of normal types

Vikings with firm connective tissue

The following advice and tips for Viking types apply to both men and women.

Stretching

You should stretch your fascia as much and as often as you can, using slow, melting stretches as well as more dynamic stretches that involve rocking and jumping. Stretch often using your body weight or with small dumbbells, and work deliberately to the limit of your elasticity.

Spring

For the 'spring' section, try to choose exercises that involve all of the different body parts, as this will help improve your coordination and agility. After doing jumping exercises, make sure you stretch out the structures you have activated.

Revive

Any activity applied to the fascia that stimulates the metabolism is especially important for you, because your connective tissue tends to become knotted.

Feel

These exercises are suitable for everyone, but more important for the Viking types.

An overview of the exercises

❶ Opening up the rib cage (page 193)

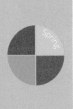 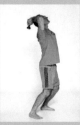 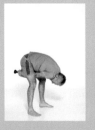

❷ Flying sword (page 194)

Other useful exercises

Other exercises that Viking types will find beneficial are 'the cat' (pp. 160/161), 'the eagle flight' (pp. 148/149), and 'swinging the legs' (pp. 180/181), as well as 'light switch Kung Fu' (page 223). These all increase flexibility and improve coordination, which is particularly important for Viking types.

 Opening up the rib cage

Men in the Viking category in particular tend to lean forward with contracted shoulders. This exercise opens the rib cage and loosens up the tight fascia in the chest.

How it works

1. Lay with your back on a foot stool, keeping your back straight so as not to form a pronounced hollow in the lower back. Take a small dumbbell or filled water bottle in each hand. Extend your arms out to the sides. Make sure that your elbow joints are always slightly bent.

2. Holding this position, let the weight of the dumbbells lower your arms until you feel a tightness across your rib cage.

3. Now start to intensify the stretch by making small, pumping movements with the arms. Make sure the motion is not a forceful snatch, but rather a comfortable spring. Vary the position of your arms on the sides and over your head by using different angles, and try different hand positions.

4. Then repeat the exercise with your arms bent.

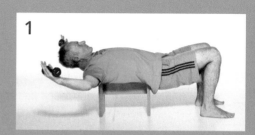

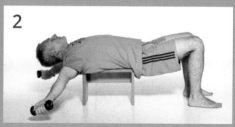

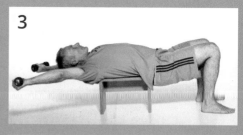

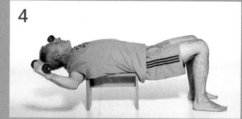

② **Flying sword**

You will already be familiar with this exercise from the short program of back exercises on pages 164 and 165. It is particular suitable for Viking types, both male and female. Please note the advice in the introduction for people with instability in their backs.

How it works

1. Hold a small 1.5 kg dumbbell (or, alternatively, a small, filled water bottle) in both hands. Raise the dumbbell up over your head. Now, start to move your upper body back and forth, making slow, snake-like movements. This pre-loads the fascia in the torso and starts to generate the momentum that you will need for the next movement. The snake-like movements should pass through the stomach and chest, and there should be movement of the thoracic spine. Do five or six repetitions of these movements while holding the dumbbell behind your head.

2. – 4. Now spring forward from your sternum. Bring your upper body down and swing your arms with the dumbbell passing backward between your legs and then back up over your head. Straighten your arms naturally into the swing. Do this smoothly and gently.

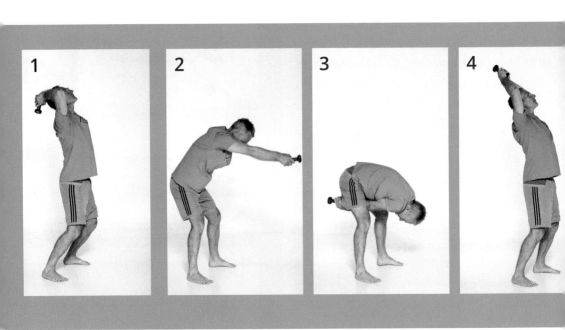

Contortionists with soft connective tissue

Stretching

It is not advisable to stretch too far or too hard. Instead, keep the range of movement during the stretching exercises small and controlled, and try to make small, deliberate changes in each position to re-train your proprioceptive awareness in your joints. For contortionists, the objective is not to become more flexible, or increase the range of motion, but rather to develop an awareness of the joints and tissue and of what the limits are. We should avoid straining in the extreme ranges of the joints.

Spring

Be cautious about practicing dynamic springy movements. To build up healthy tissue tension, it is more effective to contract the muscles in a position where the muscles you are working with are shortened to the maximum. You can tell this by the fact that these muscles are maximally thickened in the position you are aiming for. Such isometric contractions in the shortened state promote an increase in tissue tonicity.

Revive

When we are trying to revive or rejuvenate the tissue, small, fast and jerky rolling movements are beneficial, as they stimulate the connective tissue cells to increase collagen production.

Feel

Exercises from the 'feel' section are particularly important. It is common for contortionists to find that their sense of internal perception deteriorates and becomes less precise when they attempt extreme stretching positions. You should therefore actively refine your inner perception and body control over the full range of motion.

For the chest and shoulders: firming the bust

How it works

1. This exercise is good for women with soft connective tissue who want to achieve a firmer bust. Kneel on all fours, making sure that your hips are in line with your knees and your the shoulders are directly over your wrists. Keep your hands flat on the mat and press your fingertips into the floor a little. This should automatically rotate your forearms into the correct position, with the insides of your elbows facing one another.

2. Next, gently rotate your upper arm outward a little bit. Stabilise the position of your lower abdomen and lift one hand off the mat. Take a dumbbell or cuff weight in this hand and pass it sideways under your supporting arm, through to the other side. In this extreme position practice some slow mini-bounces with your free arm towards the ceiling until exhaustion. This will strengthen the sheaths of connective tissue around your chest muscles. Then switch sides.

Tip: The exercises for women on pages 200 to 203 are also ideal for contortionist types (including men).

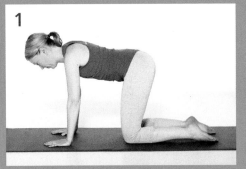
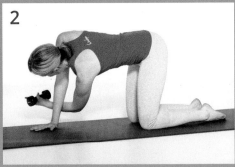

Crossover types

Stretching

The shortened regions typically found in individuals of this type – such as the back of the legs, lower back, upper chest area – should be stretched regularly.

Spring

After exercises from the 'spring' section, it is important to have another quick stretch of the areas mentioned above.

Revive

Use slow, rolling movements to rejuvenate these problem areas on the back of the legs, lower back, upper chest and neck.

Feel

These exercises are always beneficial, especially for the lower back.

Loosen up shortened areas

You should try to make a habit of stretching out the back of your calves – ideally on a step as shown on page 190 (stretching the Achilles tendon) or on another stable surface. The more slowly you do this, the more effective it will be. Try to make stretching part of your usual routine. Personally, I like to stretch my calves during short phone calls or when I'm brushing my teeth.

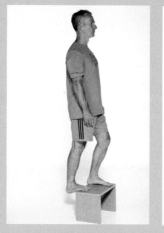
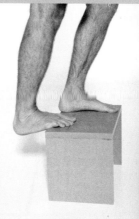

Stretching the Achilles tendon

You will also find it beneficial to roll out your lower back at the end of the day – and it feels good, too. You may find it helpful to prop your back up so that you can control how much weight you apply to the roller. Alternatively, you can rest your shoulders on the floor and lift your bent legs into the air. This will put more weight onto the lower back. Two to three minutes of this exercise, keeping your breath relaxed, can work small miracles, both for preventing back pain and improving your posture.

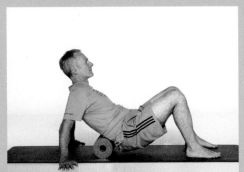 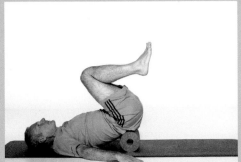

Rolling out the lumbar fascia

The 'opening up the rib cage' exercise (page 193) also works well for crossover types. In addition to exercises designed to loosen the tissue, we also recommend movements that have a strengthening and stimulating effect on the areas that tend to be weaker, such as the thighs and bottom. See the 'tightening the thighs and buttocks' exercise on page 202, for example.

Different exercises for men and women

Research and experience have demonstrated that men and women have different problem areas and want to train and shape them in specific ways. However, the evidence would suggest that the basic principles of fascia training actually apply to members of both sexes, as the connective tissue has the same set of functions in everybody. There are no fundamental differences between the two sexes, except that women naturally have slightly softer connective tissue.

The exercises in our basic program are therefore well-suited to all connective tissue types and to both sexes. If the connective tissue tests indicated that you are a Viking, contortionist or crossover type, you will find guidelines for your specific tissue type in the section above. The following exercises aim to address some typical problem areas and needs for women and for men.

Exercises and tips for women

Many women have soft tissue and cellulite in their thighs, while also suffering from tension in the neck. If this is the case for you, then we need to be focusing on exercises to strengthen and firm the thighs, along with exercises to loosen the neck area. Those dreaded dents and little rolls that often accumulate in the thigh are not something we can usually combat with muscle training alone, because the problem is caused by a lack of elasticity in the superficial fascia that runs along the outside of the thigh to just below the knee. In individuals with a certain genetic predisposition, visible fat deposits and water retention develops in this layer of fascia, which is what we see from the outside as cellulite.

However, regular fascia training improves the elastic tension in the layers surrounding the thigh; this can help to reduce or even eliminate the dimpling. Another exercise for the thighs that is really easy to fit around your daily routine is the stair dance (page 222).

An overview of the exercises

   ① Rolling out the thighs (page 201)

   ② Tightening the thighs and buttocks (page 202)

   ③ Tightening the tummy (page 203)

① Rolling out the thighs

How it works

1. Follow the instructions for the 'rolling out the outer thighs' exercise on page 177.

2. – 4. This time, however, work over your entire thigh with the roller – the outside, the front, the back and the inner thigh, as well as the section where the thigh meets the buttock.

Note: Try to make the rolling movement as slow as possible, as if in slow motion. Think of it like a sponge that you want to squeeze as much liquid out of as possible, so that it can soak up plenty of nice, fresh water.

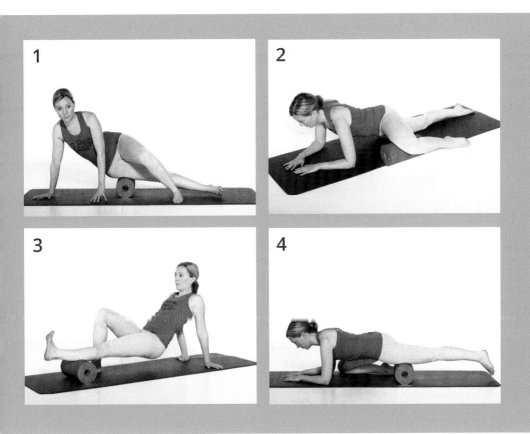

(2) Tightening the thighs and buttocks

This exercise is similar to the 'activating the outer thigh' exercise on pages 178 and 179, except this time we will work on both the inside and the outside of the thigh, and you will be lying on a chair from the start. This stimulates the fascia even more intensively. If you have problems with your wrists, shoulders or neck, making the position on the chair difficult for you, then you can perform the exercise on your side on the floor.

Ankle weights are ideal for this exercise, so it is worth investing in some. For women, an ideal weight to begin with is about 0.75 kg per cuff, but you can of course use heavier weights if you prefer.

How it works

1. Lie sideways on the chair, working the upper leg first and then the lower leg. Tense the thigh from the outside and the inside, pulling it nice and tight.

2. Then stretch out your leg like a telescope, hold this position and pulsate upwards with small, springy movements. This tightens the superficial tissue and helps to give the thigh a nice, taut appearance. Finally, repeat the exercise again, but without the ankle weight, and enjoy the light and airy feeling in your legs.

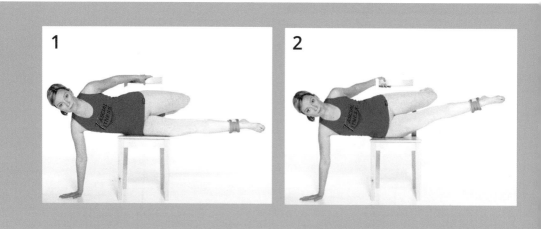

Tightening the tummy

How it works

1. Sit upright on the floor or mat, with your legs slightly apart and your feet flat on the floor in front of you. Stretch your arms forward while making sure that your shoulders stay pulled down, as if someone is pulling you forward by your fingers and simultaneously pushing a weight down on your shoulder blades.

2. + 3. Next, tilt your pelvis backward, pull your abdominal muscles slightly inward, and roll yourself about halfway down. Make sure that your abdomen remains flat and that your back is rounded. Now start to make little changes in the angle of the position, tilting a little to the right, then to the left, and rotating your upper body. Then, roll down a little lower and come up higher, making the transition between these positions as fluid as possible. Now and then, hold the position you are in and bounce gently upward.

Note: Check that you're not using too much force and have a rest if it becomes too difficult to hold your tummy in or keep your back rounded.

Variation: You can also try doing this exercise with a balloon or ball between your knees during this exercise. Press lightly on the balloon or ball throughout the exercise. This helps to tighten the pelvic floor muscles.

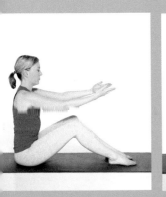

2

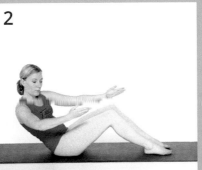

3

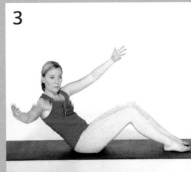

Exercises and tips for men

Men often have shortened structures in their legs, hips and shoulders, which can also be due to a lack of balance in their fitness regime. Men often want to look as toned and muscular as possible – but you should really try to avoid being so muscular that you can barely walk. Performance athletes, who focus all their efforts on just one type of sport, need to make sure that they balance this out with adequate stretching of the body parts they train so intensively; otherwise this can impact their flexibility. This is especially true for those who want to have a strong upper body and broad shoulders. Some exercises for men for improving elasticity, firmness and suppleness are given below.

An overview of the exercises

1 The flamingo (pp. 205/206)

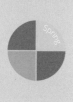 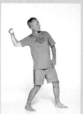 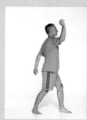

2 Throwing (page 207)

3 Stretching the adductors (pp. 208/209)

(1) The flamingo

How it works

1. Stand in front of a chair with your legs hip-width apart. Shift your weight to one side and place your free leg on the seat. Your standing leg should be stable, so make sure your knee is not completely locked.

2. Now bend your upper body forward with your arms stretched out over the leg that is resting on the chair. Keeping the knee of this leg slightly bent, bend as far forward as you need to feel a noticeable stretch in the back of the thigh. Throughout the exercise, you should maintain this amount of tension in the leg that is resting on the chair.

3. – 5. Now try varying the tension by gently shifting the stretch towards the inner leg and then towards the outer leg. Notice how this feels in the muscle chain at the back of your leg, which is often shortened. Vary the stretch with small extension and flexing movements of the knee joint. Your stretches should be cat-like and supple. Pay attention to your upper body: pull the tips of your shoulder blades slightly back and down, and keep your sternum relaxed and open throughout the leg stretch.

6. + 7. Those who are more advanced can take the exercise one step further and work on opening up this muscle group from the other end, too – starting at the pelvis. To do this, experiment with small upper body or pelvis movements. This will work on the chain of fascia that runs down the back of the leg to the feet. Take your arms forward or to the sides, and pull yourself up in the opposite direction. Try to follow your own impulses as you move and stretch – from small to large or from simple to more complex connections. This is a playful and gentle way to stretch out the entire rear chain.

Note: Because it rotates your upper body, this exercise is also very good for the back ('A short program for back problems', pp. 157–167).

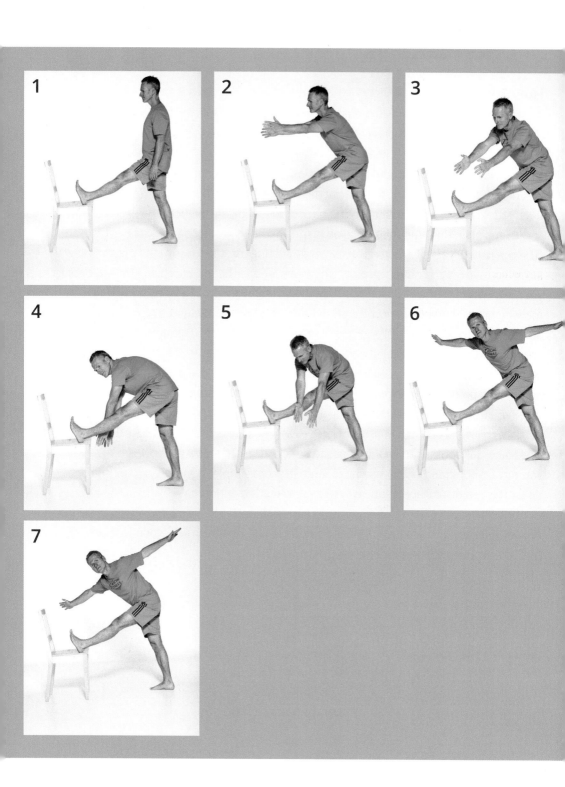

(2) Throwing

  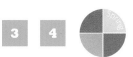

How it works

1. In this exercise you simulate a throwing motion, as if you were throwing a ball or a javelin. Try the process of performing a fluid throwing motion without too much force. It is important to pre-load the torso and arm structures like a rubber band through a counter-movement in preparation for the throw. You can hold a ball or convenient object in your hand, without actually throwing it. This activates the brain pattern of movement during practice.

2. – 3. Lean back slightly and pull your arm back in preparation for the throwing action. At this point, the stored energy can be used without much force being necessary for projectile motion. You do not really need to throw anything – it's all about tension and stimulus. Make sure that the throwing movement impulse comes from the shoulder, and not from the hand like a whipping action. The movement is initiated by the set-up in the shoulder, but then the hand follows through effortlessly like the end of a whip. This exercise is also part of our short program of exercises for the back (pp. 157–167).

Advanced variation: Lead the movement with your sternum and let it flow gradually through the shoulder and arm, and then to the hand.

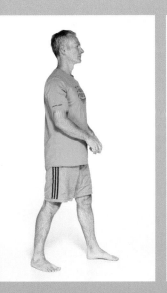

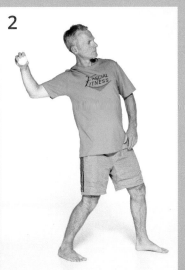

2

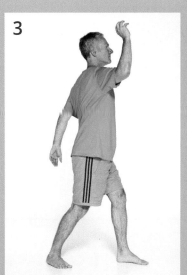

3

③ **Stretching the adductors**

How it works

1. This exercise focuses on the inner thighs. The muscles there are called the adductors. Start by taking a step out to the side. In this position, perform gentle rocking movements with your outstretched leg.

2. Next, transfer the support of the extended leg to the heel and rotate the foot outward. From here make rocking, springing movements with your upper body in different directions.

3. Now turn the extended leg completely inward, so that the foot rests on the instep. Stretch the opposite arm over the body and back so that the upper body twists slightly. In this position, experiment with slow stretches. Enjoy playing about with different movements, and trying little rocking springs while your leg is stretched out as far as it will go. You will find it very helpful to practice mindful breathing while doing this exercise. You can find tips on how to do this on pages 139 and 141.

4. – 6. Practice all three parts of the exercise on different areas of your body to stimulate the fascial network as effectively as possible.

Note: The 'opening up the rib cage' exercise, described in the section for Viking types on page 193, is also really good for men – especially those whose work involves sitting in a hunched position and who do not tend to compensate for this during their free time. Contrary to popular belief, conventional strength training does not make the body more stiff, but – generally speaking – makes it more flexible! That isn't to say that it's going to turn you into a ballerina or a master yogi, but you will be significantly more mobile with strength training than without.

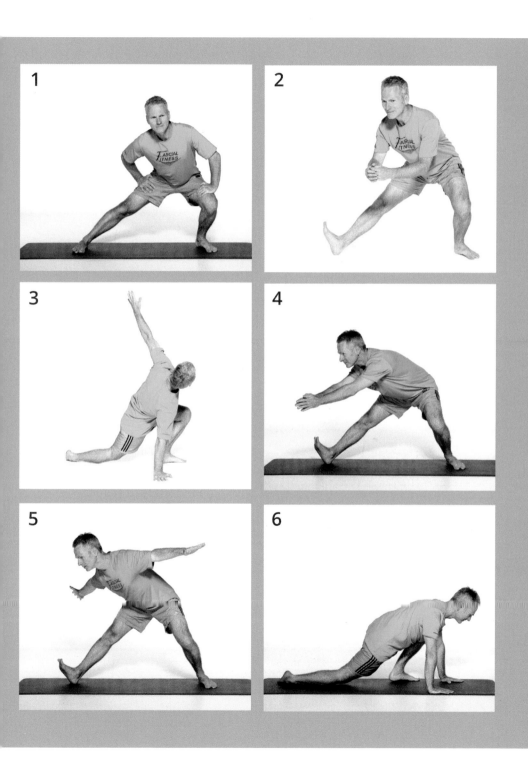

Exercises for athletes

Athletes are by definition well trained, yet they are still susceptible to certain problems, including restricted movement and pain. These conditions often occur as a result of unbalanced training as well as injuries or excessive strain. New knowledge and research regarding fascia has contributed a better understanding in recent years, including about the involvement of the fascia in sore muscles, and the realisation that connective tissue in good condition helps prevent injuries. In the majority of sports injuries, it is the white fascia that is affected and not the muscles. What has also had a strong impact is new knowledge about the elastic storage capability of fascia, which is drawn on in various forms of training.

In certain sports, some fascial and muscular problems occur very often. In this section, we will address a few of the most common ones. If you want to delve more deeply into this subject, take a look at the sports science literature recommended in the Appendix.

Special tips for athletes
- ▶ Sport-specific fascial care (page 211)
- ▶ Self-help for muscle soreness (pp. 212–216)
- ▶ Balancing exercises for runners (pp. 217–219)
- ▶ Tips for cyclists (page 220)

Sport-specific fascial care

Flexibility is important for all athletes, though for some more than others. It is our collagen structures, rather than the contractile muscle fibres, that affect how flexible we are. The fascial tissue – the tendons, ligaments, muscle sheaths and joint capsules – has to be maintained, and the appropriate fascia training is a must for athletes. It is essential to do regular exercises that stimulate these tissues and increase your muscle perception.

Begin each training session for your sport with the fascia exercises from the revive section, such as rolling out the structures that you use the most, be it the thighs, calves, feet or back. Before you train, you can roll out the muscles at a slightly faster pace. This stimulates and increases our sense of our own movements, otherwise known as proprioception.

Depending on their sport, each athlete will have a different area they need to focus on and should pick the exercises that correspond to those areas.

Rolling out after training, after intense exercise and after competitions is different. In these instances, roll very slowly. Slowly rolling out the tissue is relaxing and stimulates tissue regeneration. For tips on how to do this, see the exercises in the next section on muscle soreness. We also recommend the following two programs:

▶ A short program for back problems (pp. 157–167)
▶ The hip area (pp. 176–182)

Anyone who does strength training should always stretch the trained areas of muscle sufficiently to compensate for muscle tightening and maintain their flexibility. For golfers, tennis players and participants in other ball and racket sports, the elastic storage capacity of the tendons in the shoulders and arms is particularly important. The throwing exercise on page 207 is good for this.

Self-help for muscle soreness

Here we have put together a short self-help program for muscle soreness, comprising of slow stretching and rolling out fascia using a roller. The rolling-out is like a self-massage. A real massage would be even better, of course, but for most people that's a bit of a luxury. So grab your roller and do it yourself! Adjust the pressure as you roll – it should not feel overly painful, but rather you should get that comfortable 'good pain' we have talked about in the sore tissue.

Slow, gentle stretches are also really good for muscle soreness, such as the 'elephant step' (page 216) and exercises like 'the cat' (pp. 160/161), 'the flamingo' (pp. 205/206) or the 'eagle flight' (pp. 148/149). On the next few pages, you will find recommendations for more stretching exercises relating to specific areas of soreness.

An overview of the exercises

 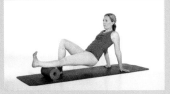   ① Rolling out the calves (page 213)

 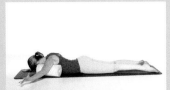   ② Rolling out other parts of the body to relieve muscle soreness (pp. 214/215)

 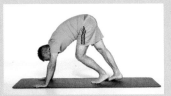   ③ Slow stretching for muscle soreness: elephant step (page 216)

Rolling out the calves

This exercise helps to alleviate muscle aches in the calves. It is also good for runners, skiers and cyclists, who often have shortened, over-trained calf muscles.

How it works

1. Sit comfortably on the floor. Place you hands on the floor behind you to support your upper body. Make sure that your shoulder girdle stays nice and stable and that your head does not sink down between your shoulders. Position the roller at the base of one calf, about level with the Achilles tendon. Bend the knee of the other leg to give you more control over the amount of pressure you apply. Lift your bottom off the floor, and slowly and carefully begin to put weight onto the contact point. Then let the roller slowly make its way up the calf, millimetre by millimetre, by moving the contact point slowly and gently. Do this exercise as if in slow motion. If the pressure is too painful, then keep your pelvis on the mat.

2. If you want to increase the pressure, you can add extra weight by placing your other leg on top of the leg that is on the roller.

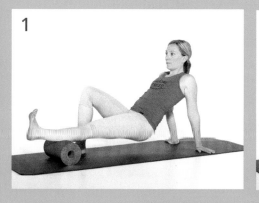
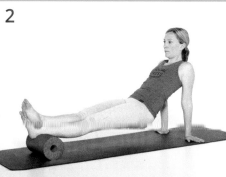

② Rolling out other parts of the body to relieve muscle soreness

This slow, relaxing rolling exercise can be done with several different parts of the body, including the thighs and back. You can also use balls or smaller rollers to roll out the forearms, chest and upper body. Here is an overview:

1. Rolling out the chest muscles and fascia with a tennis ball

2. Rolling out the chest and arms with a fascia roller

3. Rolling out the back and lumbar spine (pp. 158/159)

4. Rolling out the outer thighs (page 177) and rolling out the whole thigh (page 201)

5. Rolling out the front of the thigh (page 201)

6. Rolling out the back of the thigh – plus a variation with one leg placed on top of the other. This applies more pressure to the bottom leg, if that is what you want. Only apply as much pressure as you find comfortable

7. + 8. You can roll out the forearms using a small fascia roller or a filled water bottle (pp. 172/173).

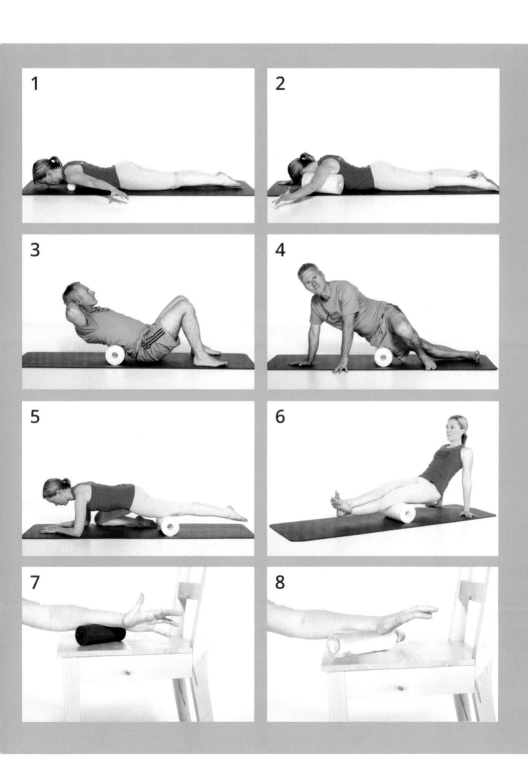

③ Slow stretching for muscle soreness: elephant step

How it works

1. Start on all fours. Make sure that your hips are over your knees and that your shoulders are over your wrists. Place your hands flat on the mat and press your fingertips slightly into the floor. This will automatically rotate your forearm into the correct position, with the insides of your elbows facing one another. Next, rotate the humerus gently outward. Tighten the lower abdomen and lift your bottom into the air to create a nice, stretched triangle position. Then bring the pelvis all the way back down, and lower your heels as far as possible toward the mat.

2. Now bend your knees one after the other, as you did in the cat exercise (pp. 160/161), and push the opposite sit bone even further into the air.

3. + 4. Gradually creep your hands, step by step, up towards your feet. As you do this, your bottom will rise even higher, and the angle formed by your body will become more acute. Once you find that you cannot get your hands any closer to your feet, walk your hands forward, step by step, until you return to the starting position.

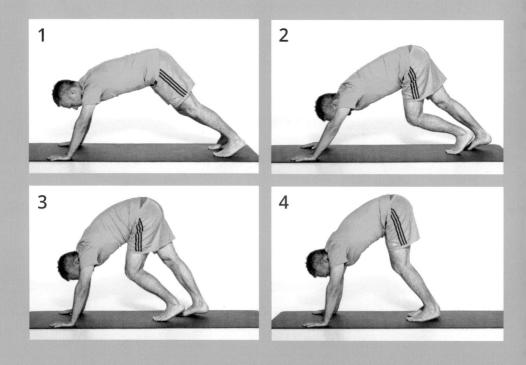

Balancing exercises for runners

It is important for runners to stretch the heavily stressed Achilles tendon in order to keep it supple and to increase elasticity and capacity for storing kinetic energy. The stretching exercise that uses a bench or step is particularly good for the Achilles tendon.

Otherwise, the best advice I can give to runners is to keep their training as varied as possible. Endurance runners in particular move in a very uniform fashion, with a limited set of movements. It is therefore beneficial to change the movement pattern every now and then.

If you are an endurance runner, i.e. you run more than 5000 metres at a time, I recommend that you take short breaks in the run from time to time. This protects the fascial structures in the legs from the main problems that tend to affect runners. For example, you can try switching from running to walking for 30 seconds – taking long strides – when you are a quarter of the way through your run, then another at the halfway point, and then after three quarters.

If you have good body awareness, you can practice taking little walking breaks like this as and when you notice that you aren't running with quite the same energy and vigour. When this happens, the flight phases become shorter and you no longer land quite as softly on your feet. If you take short walking breaks at the right intervals, you will notice that your fascia regains its elastic storage capacity in the first few strides following the break. The interesting thing here is that, as recent studies have shown, most runners who take these short walking breaks actually arrive at the finish line just as quickly as they would without taking any breaks at all.

An overview of the exercises

1 Stretching the Achilles tendon (page 218)

2 Running variations (page 219)

Stretching the Achilles tendon

You will already be familiar with this exercise from the program 'For the feet and gait' on page 190. Take note of the advice specified there. Here's a brief reminder of the exercise.

How it works

1. Stand on a stool. Pull back one heel a little and let it float freely, while keeping the other foot flat on the stool.

2. Now push the floating heel down and hold this position for a few moments. Then vary the position of the heel using small angle changes to achieve a stretch in the various fibres.

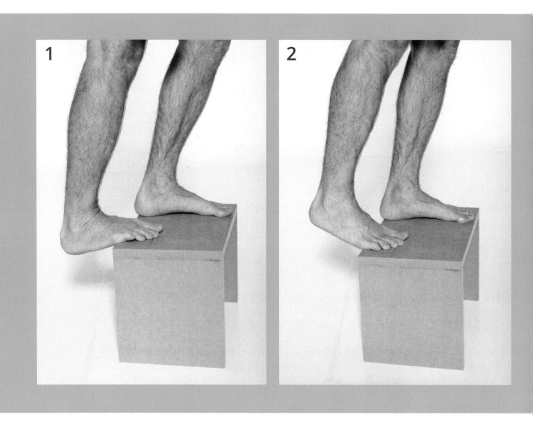

(2) **Running variations**

How it works

1. + 2. Try changing directions – running backwards or sideways. Try crossing your legs over one another like a grapevine, and build in a few hops here and there.

Variations: Benches, tree roots and pavements also offer the perfect opportunity for a bit of variation. Jump up onto them and back down again, landing softly as you do. Keep your movements lively and agile, so that you can train your body awareness and fascia while running at your best. This also subjects your joints and tendons to a greater variety of load angles.

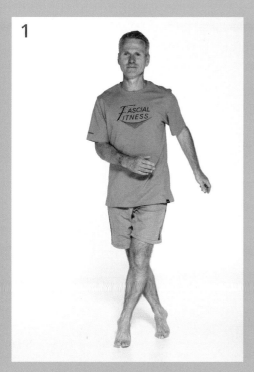

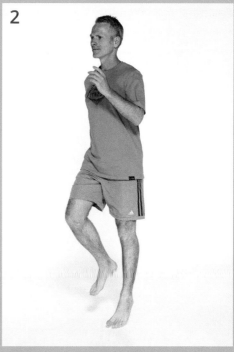

Tips for cyclists

Cyclists tend only to use very specific parts of the body when riding – namely the calves, thighs and hips. The movement sequence is always the same, and the strain on the knees and hip joints falls within a very small radius. The backs of the thighs are often shortened in cyclists, and the structures above the knees and the hips are sometimes less mobile. In my experience, competitors in the Tour de France and other long cycling races suffer for quite a few days after the event. They become extremely stiff, which is probably because of the one-sided strain.

Therefore, if you only train specific muscles for your sport, it is not just that particular muscle group that is affected, but also the entire musculofascial unit. This is mainly because of swelling – or, specifically, fluid congestion – in the connective tissue around the muscle. Over time, unbalanced training can actually shorten the muscle tissue.

Cyclists should therefore intentionally compensate for this by regularly performing stretching exercises, such as 'the cat' (pp. 160/161) and the 'eagle flight' (pp. 148/149). The 'opening up the rib cage' exercise (page 193) also works well because cyclists often have their upper bodies bent right over as they ride. This tends to cause uneven use of the large dorsal line, especially over long routes and long periods of intensive training. This results in strain and shortening of the fascial line down the back of the thigh to just below the knee, as well as in the back of the neck, while the entire back area is continually overstretched.

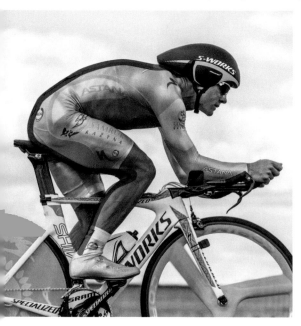

Uneven load: in cyclists, the long fascial line that runs down the back of the body is shortened in some places and overstretched in others.

Everyday life as an exercise: making your movements more creative

Our top tip for moving more creatively in your day-to-day life: use your full range of motion – make all your movements more varied and more playful! This will challenge and stimulate your fascia and utilise your joints more comprehensively. It will also help you move in a way that is more natural to your body, and keep your musculoskeletal system healthy without the need to take up a specific sport or fitness regime.

The exercises below are things you can do while simply going about your everyday life. You don't even need to wear gym clothes. Of course, you probably shouldn't try light switch Kung Fu when you're in the office or at a friend's place, so maybe save that one for when you're at home. But if your boss isn't in, you can do the 'stair dance' on the steps at work, or even do a few African bends in the office when you're picking up a paper clip. The stair dance is a great way to tighten fascia in your thighs and it is virtually effortless. Plus, it is far more effective than dodgy cellulite rollers or questionable firming creams. For the best results, try to do the stair dance two or three times a week for just a few minutes each time – but make sure you leave at least 48 hours in between.

An overview of the exercises

   ① Stair dance (page 222)

   ② Light switch Kung Fu (page 223)

   ③ African bends in everyday life (page 224)

(1) Stair dance

How it works

Every step you come across is another opportunity for a little fascia exercise! Spring from one step to the next, landing as softly as you can, and varying the position of the foot as you land. Turn inward and outward, and jump to the right and left of the stairs, as well as up and down, keeping the movements controlled and quiet.

Note: This 'stair dance' can be done with bare feet or while wearing shoes, in gym clothes or in whatever you happen to have on at the time. However, please don't do it wearing high heels, as you need the soles to be flexible. The movements should feel a bit like a dance. Make them playful and easy – it shouldn't feel like hard work. Ideally, you should get into the habit of doing this on every step.

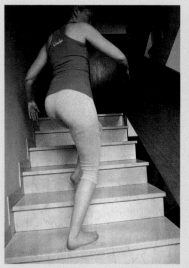
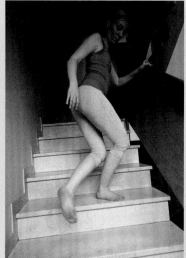
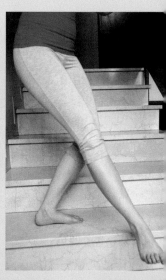
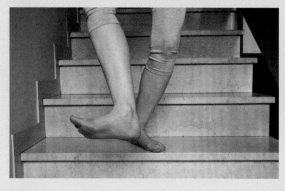
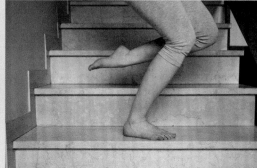

(2) Light switch Kung Fu

You will need a little confidence for this exercise, but you can really have fun doing it. It will make you feel like the Karate Kid or a masterful Kung Fu fighter. The trick is to try and turn the light on and off with your foot rather than using your hands. Of course, it isn't ideal to do this while wearing dirty outdoor shoes, especially since you will probably hit the wall a few times when you first start.

How it works

1. Focus on the light switch, take a step to the side and get ready to kick with your back foot.

2. Then aim your chosen foot at the switch, swing your foot up and – with a little luck – flick it on. More advanced Light Switch Kung Fu masters can also try turning and hitting the switch with their back to the wall.

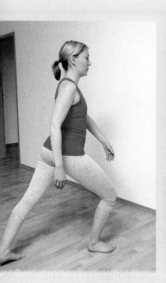
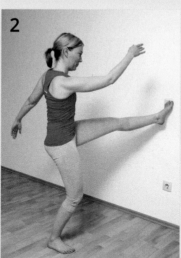
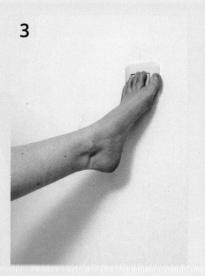

(3) African bends in everyday life

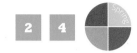

Any time you have to pick something up off the floor, you can have a quick practice of the swinging bends described on pages 162 and 163, by springing deeply out of the lumbar region while in the bend. As you do this, use the whole range of movement and bounce your upper body once or twice.

The same caution applies here: Some people can naturally keep their backs straight when doing these sorts of exercises (1), while others find their spine is naturally more rounded (2). This largely depends on how flexible you are. However, the main thing to focus on here is to activate that elastic, springing movement – not to keep a straight back.

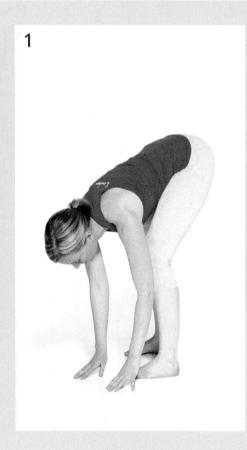

1

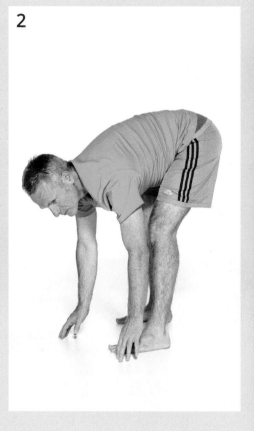

2

Guidelines for the elderly

Ageing changes fascia, especially since many older people become less active over time. 'If it sits, it sticks!', so to speak. For older people, fascia training is therefore particularly important. Here are some tips specifically for people over the age of 60.

- ▶ Regeneration of the connective tissue takes a little longer as you get older. Regular rolling and stimulating the fascia with exercises from the 'revive' section stimulates the fascia's metabolism and helps to maintain the tissue.
- ▶ In everyday life, flexibility and coordination are particularly important for maintaining our general mobility and avoiding falls, for example. So choose plenty of exercises from the 'stretch' and 'feel' sections.
- ▶ When it comes to the strengthening exercises referred to in the 'spring' section, try to pick ones that use whole body momentum and improve coordination. Although you do not need to generate an excessive amount of power, you should still exercise with greater care. Here you will find two exercises that are particularly good for this: swinging bamboo and flying sword.

An overview of the exercises

 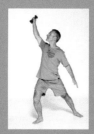

1 Swinging bamboo (page 226)

 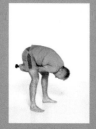

2 Flying sword (page 227)

Swinging bamboo

You will already be familiar with this exercise from the 'Exercises for problem areas' section. Here's a brief overview to jog your memory. For the full description of the exercises, take a look back at pages 174 and 175.

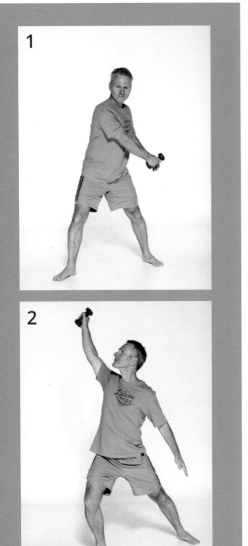

How it works

1. Assume a stable standing position like a Sumo wrestler. Your legs should be slightly further than hip-width apart, with the tips of your toes pointing outwards slightly. Your knees should be slightly bent, so that they extend just beyond the tips of your toes. Make sure that your back is straight and there is not a pronounced curve in the small of your back. Holding the dumbbell with both hands in front of your body, start by swinging it in small circles around the spinal chain. This will gradually warm up the fascia. Perform these circle swings for about a minute.

2. Then, swing diagonally up and back to one side for a few repetitions, before adding in your legs. To do this, bend your knee on the side you are swinging towards, straightening your other leg. Try opening your arms as you swing. When you swing to the right, let go of the dumbbell with your left hand. Swing with your right arm, with the dumbbell in your hand, diagonally upward to the right, and rotate the torso up to the right. Remain in this position for a moment. Now use the momentum from the bounce to spring back down again: stretch out the whole of your side in an arch shape, and swing diagonally back down, leading with the chest area.

② **Flying sword**

You will also be familiar with this exercise from the 'Exercises for problem areas' section. Here's a brief overview to jog your memory. For the full description of the exercise, take a look back at pages 164 and 165. The 'flying sword' is a great exercise for your whole body, but do make sure you do it carefully. Start very gently and try to avoid any sudden or jerky movements. Use your breath to set the pace of the movement.

How it works

1. Take a small 1.5 kg dumbbell in each hand. Raise the dumbbell up over your head. Next, start to move your upper body forward and backward, in slow snake-like movements; this brings the body's fascia into play and generates the momentum. The snake-like movements should pass through the stomach and chest, and there should be movement of the thoracic spine. Do five or six repetitions of these movements while holding the dumbbell behind your head.

2. Now spring forward from your sternum. Bring your upper body down and swing your arms with the dumbbell passing backward between your legs and then back up over your head. Straighten your arms naturally into the swing. Do this smoothly and gently. Swing six or seven times, from top to bottom and back again.

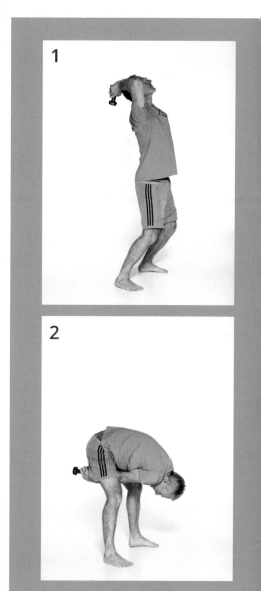

Chapter 4

ascia, physiotherapy and gentle methods of recovery

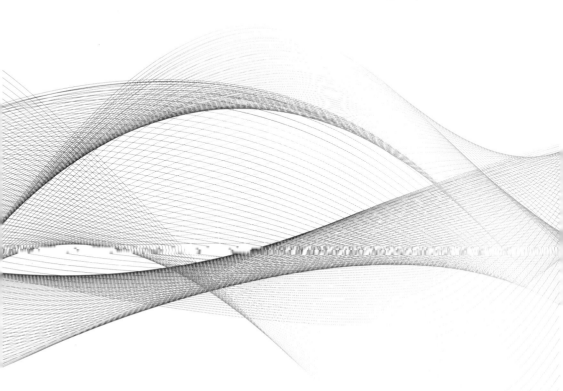

There is a close connection between fascia, physiotherapy and several methods of movement and recovery. Just how close this connection is has only been recently discovered – through the latest fascia research. Physiotherapy is possibly the field in which the new findings have the most gravitas, with entire theories and methods potentially now needing to be completely reconsidered. Physiotherapists at various levels are also fascia specialists – in 2007, at the first international Fascia Congress at Harvard University, invitations were extended to physiotherapists in addition to physicians and biologists. Throughout their years of experience with the body and the way it responds to touch and manual therapy, physiotherapists have accumulated a wealth of observations that can be of huge benefit to fascia research. My own training as a Rolfing therapist and Feldenkrais teacher fills me with enthusiasm for the scientific side of this work.

In this chapter, I would like to explain some of the implications of the new findings gained from fascia research, when it comes to manual and other so-called 'alternative' procedures. I find this area very interesting and it has opened up several avenues to integrative therapies. The procedures I am talking about include manual therapy and massage, as well as various other movement theories and even a few more recent trends. Human understanding of the healing effects of movement and touch goes back a long, long time. It is likely that the origins of the remedial use of gymnastics and massage go back as far as the Stone Age, with various forms found in many cultures all over the world. There have been records of physical exercises and manual therapy in China, which has one of the oldest sporting cultures in the world, from the 4th millennium BC. Practices from India, which has one of the oldest traditions of systematic medicine in the world, date just as far back. There, folk medicine includes elements of gymnastics and massage to this very day. In European medicine and culture, especially that of ancient Greece and Rome, there have been strong traditions of physical exercise and massage, both in sport and in the art of healing. The fact that massage has a calming effect and promotes healing has been medically confirmed.

This knowledge became somewhat neglected in the European Middle Ages, but made a comeback during the Renaissance, and truly blossomed after the Age of Enlightenment. In the 19th century especially, there was almost a continental movement in physical education, with major influences from Friedrich Ludwig Jahn – the 'father of German gymnastics'. Manual procedures were extensively promoted during this period through natural medicine, which was particularly prevalent in Germany during this time. A second wave occurred from the 1920s to the 1950s. There was also a whole new boom in gentle 'Eastern' and alternative methods in the 1970s, sparking the popularity of practices like yoga, shiatsu, acupuncture, qigong, Pilates and many more.

Fascia research is now able to shed new light on the science behind the success of these different methods. We now know that many of these so-called 'gentle' or 'complementary' practices actually have genuine physiological effects that could not previously be explained. This applies to acupuncture, yoga and osteopathy, among others. The original underlying theories of life energy, meridians, blockages, or 'disturbed harmony' derived from traditional knowledge, sometimes intuitive insights and experiences, or simply speculation. Esoteric concepts, however, could not convince previously sceptical doctors and scientists – myself included. You already know my story in this regard. There were positive clinical outcomes, however, that at least gave the methods some credibility, even if there was no scientifically tenable explanation for them.

Today, we know a lot more. We can now assume that the reason these methods work is that they stretch and stimulate the fascia, promoting fluid exchange and triggering metabolic processes within the fascial tissue, which also interacts with the nervous system. Many methods of manual therapy and other forms of movement specifically access the fascia – it's just that many practitioners and theorists behind the procedures were unaware of this. This is the astounding thing about older methods in particular, in that traditional methods and those based merely on experience are often geared towards the fascia and effect real change in the fascial tissue. This is precisely the point at which we are able to begin finding scientific explanations for the successes and effects of these methods. I will explain by using some selected examples.

Yoga then and now

This ancient Indian exercise technique has been developing over many centuries. At least as far back as 700 BC, it was described in the older Upanishads, a collection of texts containing philosophical concepts of Hinduism. Originally, yoga consisted of a series of aesthetic exercises, which helped meditation by influencing the breathing rhythm. In the original, Hindu practice, yoga has a spiritual framework, and is embedded in a tradition of self-discipline and sacrifice. It is not an exercise regime as such, but rather belongs to the search for enlightenment and the desire for self-development.

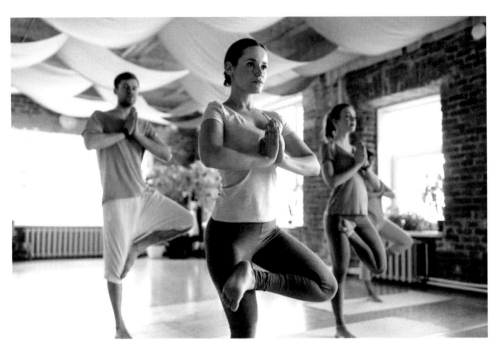

Tree pose – this seemingly ancient yoga pose is actually quite young.

The forms of yoga in the West today, however, tend to focus far more on the physical self, and are quite different from their Indian origins. That said, many of the movements and poses have remained essentially the same – whereby there has been an interesting sort of cultural exchange. Few people know that almost all of the standing poses we see in today's yoga practices do not originate from the ancient Indian tradition at all, but in fact from the European gymnastics movement of the 19th and 20th centuries. These schools, some of which we have discussed in previous chapters, were brought to India by the British army during the colonial era. Here, the soldiers would do gymnastics to keep themselves fit. Their strict fitness regimes were received with interest by the Indians, who went on to develop them further within their own system. The form of yoga practiced in India at that time consisted mainly of acrobatic contortions, tongue stretches and other exotic poses. These moves were often used by street performers to impress their crowds.

The elements of physical and sports culture imported from the West were met with great interest and were deemed to enrich the existing methods. The Indians therefore combined their age-old floor exercises with the new, lively full-body movements borrowed from the Europeans, thus creating interesting new forms of the discipline. A few decades later, in the wake of the flower power generation and Beatlemania, hoards of Westerners seeking spiritual wisdom made the pilgrimage to India. There, they would study the supposedly ancient yoga tradition and return home feeling thoroughly enlightened. What they didn't realise, however, was that it was actually a mixture of Eastern practices and Western gymnastics that they had come across.

That said, the fact that modern yoga was only developed quite recently does not detract from its effectiveness: the acknowledged success of yoga exercises in the treatment of pain, and specifically back pain, has been the subject of study by experts over the last 20 years. Yoga has been proven to reduce stress and regulate excessively high blood pressure. International scientific studies, including one from Germany by Professor Andreas Michalsen (a Berlin-based researcher of natural medicine), have confirmed these results. As far as the cause for this success is concerned, it was mainly believed in the west that yoga works by tapping into the psyche. The theory is that, because holding certain poses requires focus and perseverance, this calms the mind and reduces stress. The elements of meditation and spirituality are also deemed to be helpful, because they activate our own capacity for self-healing. It was also thought that muscle strengthening and improved circulation were responsible for the success of the discipline, and remain the basis for standard explanations of the effects of the physical elements of the practice.

Stretching helps alleviate back pain

However, yoga mainly consists of stretching exercises – specific poses that are held for a long time. This stretching obviously stimulates the fascia. It responds to this in a variety of ways, including by sending signals to the nervous system and changing tension levels. And it would seems that it is precisely this fascial response that is responsible for most of the positive physical effects – at least that's what international researchers suspect, with the work of American researcher Helene Langevin at the forefront of these findings. Helene Langevin is one of the most respected neuroscientists in the world and the Director of the National Center for Complementary and Integrative Medicine, based at Harvard University. She has used scientific methods to investigate the effectiveness and applicability of 'alternative' health treatments. In animal experiments, Langevin proved that slow stretching reduces inflammation and relieves pain. For this purpose, rats had an inflammatory substance injected into the deep fascia in their backs. The researchers were able to observe tense, cramped

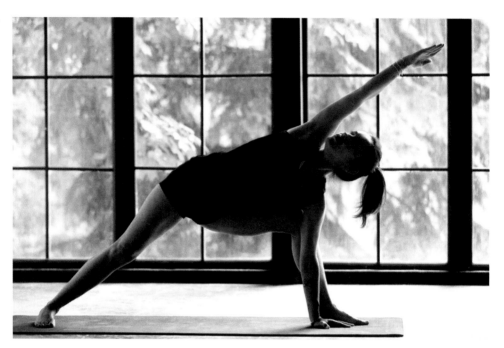

Stretching exercises like this one – a version of 'warrior pose' – are known to reduce inflammation.

movement in the animals, clearly indicating that they were experiencing back pain. Some of the rats then had their backs stretched carefully by hand for 10 minutes per day over a course of 12 days. This was designed to simulate the stretches performed during yoga practice. The result was that the rats that underwent the manual stretching recovered their normal movement, and the inflammation soon subsided. Tissue samples taken later showed that there were fewer inflammatory cells in the treated rats' lumbar fascia than in those of the untreated rats.

An extensive clinical study of back pain patients carried out by a student of Helene Langevin subsequently revealed that stretching can actually explain the benefits of yoga for these patients. A large number of patients was divided into three groups: the first took up yoga for three months, another group conducted conventional back exercises including stretching, and 45 patients read a self-help book about pain which included exercises for breathing and meditation, as well as lifestyle tips. The results showed that the group with the self-help book experienced very little benefit, whereas both the yoga and the gym exercise groups demonstrated almost the same level of success in terms of reporting less pain. This study has been documented internationally, and it is considered evidence that the pain-relieving effects of yoga are achieved not through meditation and spirituality, or even through muscle strengthening, but in fact through the slow stretching involved in the specific poses.

However, the study does not conclude what exactly it is that these stretching exercises achieve – whether it is loosening or softening of the tissue, the secretion of neurotransmitters, the transmission of signals to the autonomic nervous system or a series of proprioceptive or interoceptive phenomena. In fact, this question remains largely unanswered. Of course, more research is needed here. However, the theories about the effects of yoga on fascia and about the involvement of fascia in back pain are very convincing.

In the last few years, a new school of yoga has been growing in popularity – the branch known as 'Yin' yoga. This type of yoga involves relaxed stretching poses, held for several minutes at a time. It is possible that – in addition to the mechanical effects on the musculoskeletal system – this form of yoga can achieve a completely different set of physiological outcomes. At least, that's what recent experiments using animals and cell cultures would suggest, whereby ultra-slow stretching resulted in both reduced inflammation and accelerated wound healing. Moreover, there is a spectacular new animal experiment being carried out at Harvard Medical School in Boston. Here, researchers were able to use long stretches lasting several minutes – similar to those practiced in yoga – to drastically reduce the growth of cancerous ulcers. When I found out about this, I was absolutely fascinated and immediately got in touch with the colleagues I knew there. Of course, it is still too early to promote stretching as a reliable cancer treatment in humans, as my colleagues assured me. However, it is quite possible that, in the next few years, we will understand exactly what effects stretching has on the tissue. Until then, however, we can already conclude that ultra-slow stretching can trigger effects in the body that go far beyond improved musculoskeletal mobility.

In addition, these long stretches also seem to have a calming effect on the autonomic nervous system, which goes from a state of over-stimulation that is very symptomatic of modern life, to a state of relaxation. This calming effect has considerable reach, also affecting our blood pressure, lungs, digestion, sleep cycle, as well as heart and brain function. In the exercise chapter, we have already discussed ways in which our breathing can support this process.

For the connective tissue type of contortionists, however, ultra-slow stretching can also have negative effects, with the possibility of your joints becoming unstable if you overdo it. Therefore, if you have very soft connective tissue and your test has shown that you fall into the contortionist category, you must always exercise caution when practising intense styles of yoga. Vikings are less likely to be tempted to overstretch themselves.

Classic massage and manual therapy

As far back as the days of Ancient Greece and Rome, Olympians and gladiators would have been massaged to help recover from their sports. In fact, massage is probably the oldest healing technique in the world. So far, however, explanations for its success have been largely based on improved circulation and general loosening of the muscles. Yet, we now know that fascia plays a far more important role. Massage stimulates the metabolism in fascia, and triggers the release of neurotransmitters and hormones in the body. This is because fascia, being so close to the skin, is part of the sensory system specifically designed for social contact and human-to-human touch. Massage using a slow, rhythmic pressure also promotes the exchange of fluids in fascia, as we have already discussed. Hormones that cause stress and inflammation, as well as metabolic residues, are thus removed from the connective tissues, which then refill with fresh fluid and nutrients. As research

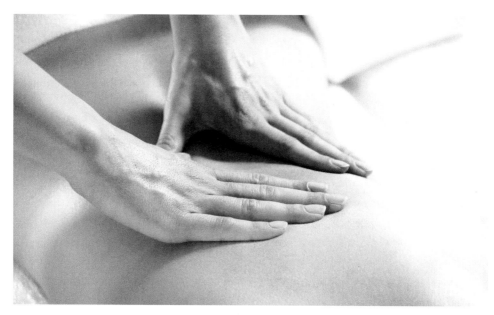

Healing methods that use the hands have their roots in ancient tradition.

has demonstrated, massage leads to the secretion of anti-inflammatory neurotransmitters in the skin and fascia. These substances can dissolve adhesions and matting in fascia. Remember the massaging of operation scars in the animal trial by Geoffrey Bove and Susan Chapelle, mentioned in Chapter 2 (page 48)? Incidentally, these animals were massaged using slow, gentle, flowing movements similar to the techniques that are applied in Rolfing therapy. The biochemical and neuroreflexive effects of massage have long been understood in the field of physiology. However, the fact that it is fascia that is so important here, rather than the muscles or just their blood and nerve supply, is a brand-new discovery.

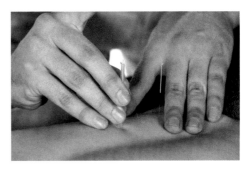

Needle therapy: acupuncture does work to alleviate pain, but not because of any mysterious energies.

energies, which can be stimulated and brought into balance through a total of 400 acupuncture points throughout the body. Very few Western researchers believe in negative energies and energetically charged meridians through which comprehensive life energy flows.

Acupuncture

Acupuncture is a complementary therapy that has been scientifically proven to help with back and knee pain. But how? The Chinese have been inserting needles into the bodies of patients since about the 2nd century BC. The theory was that life energy flows through the entire body along pathways known as 'meridians'. It is believed that, if one of these meridians becomes blocked, a needle inserted into the pathway frees the blockage. Another theory behind acupuncture involves the philosophical concepts of Yin and Yang. These are alleged to be female and male

Nevertheless, acupuncture clearly works. Again, Helene Langevin, who is researching complementary procedures, has demonstrated that fascia plays a part in this, too. The acupuncture points are located at the intersections between different sections of fascia. Here, there is a whole host of receptors which, when stimulated – whether with a needle or with pressure and massage – trigger a reflex response, sending various signals to the brain and the muscles. This is why acupuncture needles trigger responses in fascia that have a healing effect. It could also explain why studies have shown that so-called sham or placebo acupuncture also works. Here, rather than piercing the traditional acupuncture points as they are described in the literature, the researchers inject the needle slightly off to the side. However, this still stimulates areas that belong to the same sensory region – or 'dermatome', as it is known in medical terms. The fact that the same area of skin and connective tissue is stimulated could explain why sham or placebo acupuncture is also effective. Since Helene Langevin's various anatomical and physiological experiments, there has been further work in this field that has confirmed the correlation between acupuncture points and certain points of connective tissue. The Chinese now also prescribe to the belief that acupuncture works by stimulating the fascia.

Rolfing therapy

By now, you will already have some understanding of this method of manual therapy, as we covered it in our discussion of the pioneers of fascia research, and my own career. The scientific studies on Rolfing therapy have been mainly based in the US. To date, Rolfing therapy is still only recognised by a few health insurance companies, but we are working on this and are currently in the process of investigating and documenting – from a scientific perspective – the effectiveness of Rolfing for back and shoulder problems, general pain, tension and posture.

Over the years, Rolfing therapists have moved away from the original idea that Rolfing works by deforming or reshaping the connective tissue, as well as resolving any obstructions in energy flow. Ida P. Rolf was, in many respects, correct in her thinking, and was a genuine pioneer in this area, with the aim of raising the profile of connective tissue and its relationship to mobility. Some of her explanations, however, appear obsolete from today's perspective, such as the idea that, by applying enough pressure, you can permanently deform solid connective tissue. Moreover, she did not know that fascia has nerve endings, but instead regarded it as an interesting mechanical material. Had she been able to experience the rapid pace of modern fascia research, I am certain that she would be just as fascinated by the advances in our understanding as her fellow therapists are today.

After all, her insights and the gripping techniques she developed have proven to be effective. Several studies have demonstrated this, including one that was conducted over a course of ten Rolfing sessions in patients with neck pain. Rolfing techniques consist of slow, gentle massage strokes and very firm manipulation of the fascia within the muscular regions of the body such as the lumbar spine, shoulders and neck. This method also uses movement and stretching to effect change in

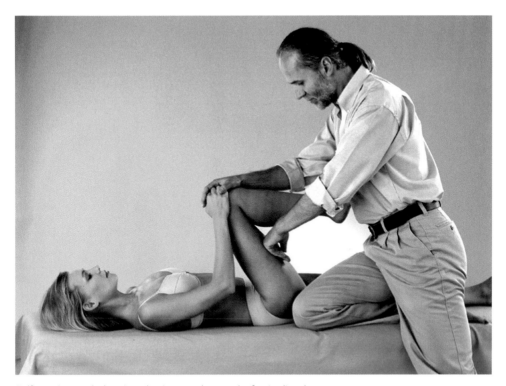

Rolfing grips reach deep into the tissue and target the fascia directly.

the shoulders and arms, as well as special grips for lifting the pelvis and thus also stimulating the long fascial lines.

Osteopathy

Osteopathy is a manual process which includes treatments for virtually all ailments. You read a little about this topic in Chapter 1 (page 51) and its founder, Andrew Taylor Still. After his death, osteopathy was further developed in different directions during the 20th century.

During this form of treatment, the therapist uses their hands to perform certain grips and massage techniques. Osteopathic treatments are somewhat controversial. However, according to studies carried out by the Osteopath Association, the treatments do work for many pain symptoms and certain regulatory problems, such as high blood pressure, migraines and chronic diseases. Osteopathy has since been accepted by some health insurance companies, although as yet neither the theoretical background nor its effectiveness has been proven, despite

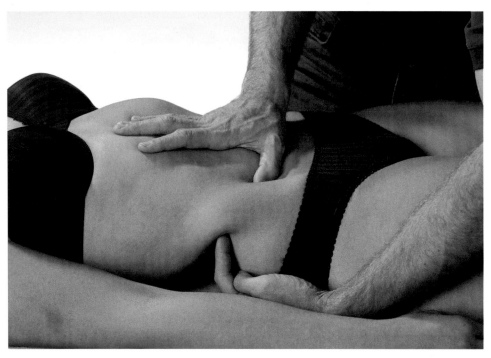

Today, osteopathic methods are heavily based on our understanding of fascia.

clearly documented research. Neverthe-less, osteopathy is very popular; it is even a university research area and forms part of medical training in the United States. The effectiveness of osteopathic treatment is currently being clinically tested.

The method is based on imagining that all the organs and parts of the body are in motion, because they are components of a living, working, fluid system. There is indeed a body-wide exchange of fluids across the fascial network; moreover, the movement of large muscles and organs is crucially dependent on smooth

functioning within their fascial sheaths. The achievements of osteopathy could be due to the manual stimulation of fascia, whereby its metabolism is in turn stimulated or neural reflexes and reactions are induced. The effectiveness of osteopathic treatments does have some scientific grounding, particularly in light of more recent findings on the role of fascia. However, there is not yet comprehensive proof of its efficacy. Osteopaths offer a solution for too many problems, and their techniques are not always consistent. However, what does seem certain is that the effectiveness of such treatment relies largely on the involvement of fascia. Some scientists, including the Italian physiotherapy researcher and osteopath Paolo Tozzi (who was also a participant of our fascia conferences), are now using the findings made in the field of fascia research to establish scientific grounds for the techniques used in osteopathy.

Pilates

The body and movement program known as Pilates was developed by a professional boxer and circus artist named Joseph Hubert Pilates, who – not by chance – had a solid sports background. He was born in 1883 in the city of Mönchengladbach in Germany, and emigrated to England in 1912, and then to the United States, where his method of training evolved into a Pilates program for soldiers and policemen. As a prisoner of war during the First World War, he used his exercises to help keep his fellow prisoners fit. Apparently, thanks to Pilates, they had a better rate of survival than many others during the great flu epidemic of 1918 to 1920. Joseph Pilates later developed his discipline to include more elements of recovery and rehabilitation, primarily as a training program for dancers. He worked on this in the United States with Rudolf von Laban, who we mentioned briefly in Chapter 3, page 77.

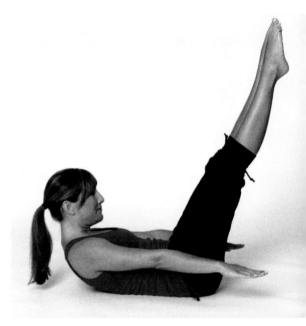

Typical Pilates exercises strengthen the body's core – like this exercise called 'the hundred'.

Pilates has become very popular because it includes dance-like and playful elements and comprises both stretching and strengthening; in particular, it improves coordination. This is not surprising, as the movements have some basis in circus acrobatics. The focus is on strengthening the core – the muscles in the abdomen, torso and pelvis – or, in Pilates speak, your "powerhouse". Strengthening this area has been shown to help with back pain. Pilates training is also an effective treatment and prevention for many other pain syndromes, as well as for stress and regulatory disorders such as high blood pressure. Pilates himself explained the effectiveness of his training through reference to 'springs' and 'bands' in the body. It is safe to assume that, being a non-medic, he was actually referring to fascia, although he did not name it specifically. He probably had an astute sense of body movement and anatomy, and hence an intuitive understanding of the participation of the fascia and fascial lines.

In check: new fascial trends

In the last few years, the range of fascia therapies and training courses has absolutely boomed. I would like to offer you some guidance in this area, which will hopefully protect you from harm and false expectations. In the table on the right, you will find a brief overview of the key trends, while the text below explains some of the more well-known methods.

The fascia distortion model (FDM)

The fascia distortion model is a method of manual therapy that was developed by the American doctor Stephen Typaldos. Having spent several years working in emergency medicine, he based his treatment on the way his patients used body language and a certain choice of words to describe their symptoms. Based on these

observations, Typaldos developed a system which identifies six specific patterns of pain and impairment. He suspected that these patterns corresponded to specific anatomical disorders, which he called 'distortions'. According to his system, the six possible types of distortion are as follows:

▶ **Trigger band:** a twisted band of fascia
▶ **Trigger point hernia:** an abnormal prolapse of tissue through the fascial sheath, such as an umbilical hernia
▶ **Continuum distortion:** an overload-induced deformation at the intersection between the bone and the tendon or ligament
▶ **Folding distortion:** a folding distortion at the muscle insertion
▶ **Cylinder distortion:** overlapping or tangling of the cylindrical coils in the superficial fascia
▶ **Tectonic fixation:** changes in the fascia's ability to glide.

Typaldos has developed specific grips designed to correct each of these disorders. Most of them are relatively painful, but they only take a few seconds and often provide immediate relief for the patient.

What is so remarkable about this method is that the diagnosis is based on the spontaneous expressions of the patient,

Name	Method	Intensity level: high (■) low (★)	Key issues	Scientific evidence
Bowen method	Gripping technique, manual	★ ★ ★	▶ Still in its infancy ▶ Practitioners are not necessarily trained therapists	A few smaller studies
Tool-based fascia treatment	Massage using special instruments	■ ■	▶ Not suitable for self-treatment ▶ Only to be performed by trained therapists	Numerous independent studies indicate a high level of effectiveness
Fascia blaster	Intense rubbing with hard plastic tool	■ ■ ■ ■	▶ Popular in Hollywood ▶ Has been the subject of several lawsuits pertaining to the obvious permanent damage to treated areas	None
Fascia distortion model (FDM)	Massage, manual	■ ■ ■ ★	▶ The majority of the grips are very painful ▶ Most effective for shoulder and arm problems	Practically none
Fascia ReleaZer	Gentle rubbing with massage roller	★ ★	▶ Ideal for controlling your breathing pattern	Several smaller studies
Self-treatment using a fascia roller	Rolling out areas of the body to promote fluid exchange	■ ■ ★ ★	▶ Ideal for self-treatment, except for a few patients (see text) ▶ Many positive effects; good for regeneration and muscle soreness	Numerous independent studies and three systematic reviews

with the therapist interpreting the patient's subconscious gestures. For example, if the injured person presses a certain point with several fingers or the thumb when describing the pain, this tells the therapist that they have a herniated trigger point – whereby the tissue bulges out from a deeper layer. On the other hand, if the patient grasps the joint with their whole hand, this apparently indicates a folding distortion – whereby there is considered to be a crease or fold in the fascial sheath.

As a trained psychologist, I am reluctant to assume that the subconscious is 'always right'. Nevertheless, I do find this method fascinating and I think it is highly likely that it does frequently direct the therapist towards the correct site and cause of the pain.

As yet, there have not been any scientific studies on the fascia distortion model. Still, it's a very interesting approach and I have seen some instances of Typaldos's treatment that appeared to be very effective. However, I am not overly convinced by the theory behind the model. It seems a little outdated to me, as it assumes that the pain is caused solely by mechanical changes in the architecture of individual layers of fascia, and does not take into account the role of other biochemical and neurological mechanisms. Also, in the many sonograms and anatomical preparations that I have seen over the years, I have only very rarely witnessed the sort of twisting and perforations described by Typaldos.

In the German-speaking world, Typaldos's model is already quite popular among athletes, and therapists swear by his corrective grips, especially in the shoulder and arm region. Caution is advised, however, especially for sensitive patients, as some FDM therapists can be particularly head-strong and the treatment can be quite rough. The following applies not just to FDM, but to any form of therapy: having the right chemistry and mutual understanding between patient and practitioner is often even more important than choosing the right method.

Bowen therapy

Bowen therapy is quite a gentle form of massage therapy, developed by the Australian Thomas Bowen in the 1950s. Bowen originally worked in a cement factory and was completely self-taught as a therapist. He later called himself an 'osteopath'. He worked purely according to his intuition and personal experience. His so-called 'Bowen moves' consist of rolling grips in which the therapist pushes the tissue across the primary grain – working on both the belly and the sinewy ends of the muscle.

Because this method is not officially recognised, either academically or scientifically, its practitioners do not always have medical or physiotherapy training. Probably thanks to the gentle, sensitive approach, this has not led to any major lawsuits or furore from the medical community. In fact, as far as we know, patients often report from personal experience that Bowen therapy has been greatly beneficial to them.

That could well be the case, and I have a very reasonable explanation as to why: it is possible that the rolling movements of the fascia and tendons stimulate the Golgi receptors, which then leads to a decrease in muscle tension. Of course, this only explains one element of the extensive and long-lasting therapeutic effect that advocates of the treatment rave about. However, the method is still quite new in Europe and, unfortunately, it has not been subject to any reliable studies. Nevertheless, Bowen therapy is enjoying increasing popularity, mostly thanks to word-of-mouth recommendations.

Trigger point therapy

I have to confess that, for a long time, I had more than a few doubts about trigger point therapy. The concept that complex pain in the soft tissue can be traced back to individual points of hardened tissue seems a little too simplistic for me. After all, that is essentially what trigger points are: hardened points in the muscle and soft tissue in certain parts of the body, which supposedly trigger problems elsewhere. I have found it difficult to believe that all you have to do is re-soften the tissue with a few determined hand grips. However, a few studies conducted in recent years have made me reconsider my stance. In fact, there do seem to be bundles of

muscle fibres that harden as if in a state of rigor mortis, and frequently so. This may be caused by long-term circulatory problems, as a result of sitting for long periods or repetitive strain, for example. When our posture or movements are heavily geared towards one side or part of the body, this leads to a lack of oxygen in the tissue and releases neurotransmitters that cause inflammation. Then, not only does the affected area become over-sensitive, but our neural circuits can also cause soft tissue pain to arise in other parts of the body, too.

The method involves using strong thumb grips to work out the trigger points. A few smaller studies have now shown that this does work, but they are yet be substantiated with larger ones. An interesting variant of the method involves the use of shock waves to points at which the pain arises. I have personally witnessed this method have a significant effect on several patients and am curious to see whether the procedure will soon be backed up with clinical evidence. The same applies to trigger point therapy using needles. This method is called 'dry needling' and is similar to acupuncture. In Germany, only doctors or certified practitioners are allowed to practice this treatment; while in Switzerland it can also be performed by specially certified physiotherapists. As in acupuncture, the

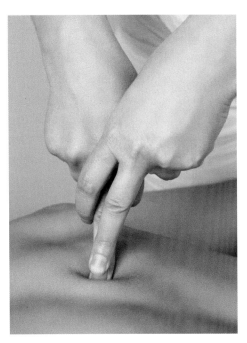

Strong pressure on trigger points can release tension.

Tools for fascial treatment

Instead of treating the hardened or matted fascia using just their hands, more and more therapists are turning to small scrapers, spoons and other instruments to help release fascial tension. I find this particularly useful when it comes to treating scar tissue, as – with a little practice – you can move more gently and slowly through the hardened areas of fibre using a tool than you could with your own fingers. Until a few years ago, most of these instruments were still made of wood, but today there are many advanced versions made of plastic and metal. Personally, I like to use the Fazer set when working on hardened scar tissue and on the heel pads. This comes in the form of a little tool case containing various differently shaped metal implements for scraping, pressing and releasing the fascia. There are also excellent fibrosis hooks and other devices available.

needles are inserted into the body, but not into the supposed 'meridians' or the actual knots in the fascia. Instead, the practitioner injects the needle directly into the myofascial hardenings identified as trigger points. This procedure came about through pure chance: doctors discovered that patients who had an anaesthetic injection administered directly into these painful lumps experienced pain relief, even if the needle did not actually contain any anaesthetic. In other words, the symptoms disappeared even if it was just the needle that was injected, with no medication at all.

There have only been a few small studies into their effectiveness in humans, but the results have been encouraging, and there are some equally positive results from animal experiments. However, caution should always be applied when using these devices on humans. That said, an experienced and well-trained fascia therapist should be able to work just as well with their tools as they can with their hands. The effectiveness of the treatment therefore depends mostly on how good the therapist is, rather than their equipment.

Fascia blasting and the Fascia ReleaZer for treating cellulite

Treatments designed to diminish cellulite – the unwanted dimples in the connective tissue just beneath the skin – are causing a real sensation, especially in the US. Promoters of so-called 'fascia blasting' recommend a particularly brutal method that claims to reduce the amount of cellulite in 'problem areas'. The idea is to rub your thighs or buttocks vigorously with a stick that has spiky appendages attached to it, until they become visibly and persistently red. The theory is that this then tightens the skin and connective tissue, with advocates of the technique proudly showing off their before-and-after photos on social media, many of which also feature some pretty significant bruising. From my perspective, the smooth surface that these photos appear to show is mainly due to temporary swelling of the underlying tissue that occurs as part of the healing of the wounds created by the device. In most cases, the smoothness does not last. There have been countless warnings and over a hundred complaints from buyers to the American health authorities, with many users having apparently incurred permanent injury from practising this brutal method. I therefore strongly recommend against this procedure and, if you do use it, I urge you to practice extreme caution.

On the other hand, I find gentle rubbing treatments, which are also available in

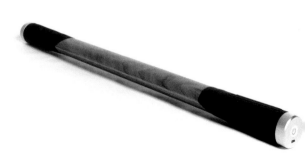

The Fascia ReleaZer from BLACKROLL uses targeted pressure to create a deeply effective vibrating massage.

Germany, far more promising. They take a much more sensitive approach to the tissue, such as the device known as the 'Fascia ReleaZer'. This vibrating wand can be used without causing severe pain or visible tissue damage.

There are also other gentle ways that you can strengthen weak areas of the body, which are also more sustainable. Regular jogging or jumping rope, for example, tightens the connective tissue, and of course I particularly recommend our own fascia exercises from Chapter 3 on page 142.

Self-treatment using a fascia roller

Fascia rolling is now practiced by many therapists and coaches, and it has been an integral part of the range of regenerative treatments used by athletes for many years. As we discussed in Chapter 2, what makes this method so effective is the fluid exchange in the tissue, which nourishes and refreshes the fascia. To create the effect you're looking for – that of squeezing out a sponge – it is important to perform the rolling movements in different directions. Specialists call this 'multi-directional' rolling. Right from the start, foam rollers have been the most widely accepted accessories for fascia treatment. Our specific brand of fascia exercises received a little more scrutiny, but even the critics soon realised that rolling out the tissue not only feels good, but has immediate effects, too.

It is quite remarkable that there have been so few reports of negative experiences or effects, especially considering that the use of these rollers is so widespread in the sports, fitness and yoga scene. Rolling is low risk and highly effective, with users seeing immediate results in terms of how well they feel. However, just to be on the safe side, please take note of the following:

► If you are healthy and have no signs of weakened venous function, rolling is absolutely fine for you. However, if you do have weak or varicose veins, thrombosis, circulatory disorders or you are taking medication to thin your blood, please consult your doctor first. This is especially true for people with weak veins. Similar to compression stockings, it is the amount of pressure on the veins that determines whether this method is beneficial or dangerous. You may need to apply more or less pressure, depending on your physiology and the type of condition you have. You should therefore consult a doctor in order to establish how much pressure to apply.

► We also have some important advice for anyone who suffers from lymph congestion in their legs: try to ensure that you are always rolling in the direction of the lymph, i.e. towards the trunk. In individuals with congestion syndromes, the tissue fluid often contains proteins and other larger cells that are too large to drain out through the small openings in the veins. We therefore need to ensure that they can drain off in the direction of the lymph.

As a general rule: To be on the safe side, you should never roll beyond your initial pain threshold. In other words, any pain you feel should be 'good pain'.

The positives outweigh the negatives
So we have looked at the potential drawbacks; now what about the positives?

There is in fact scientific research to suggest that rolling is good for the health of our blood vessels. For example, a more recent study from 2014 showed that after rolling, the test subjects had an increased concentration of nitric oxide in their blood plasma. Nitric oxide relaxes the blood vessels and makes the vessel walls more elastic. It also prevents the platelets from clumping and therefore helps the blood to flow better. The scientists responsible for this study concluded that self-massage using a roller could be a suitable method for making the arteries more supple and improving the function of the vascular wall.

This observation is particularly helpful when it comes to the question of whether rolling treatment is suitable for people with weakened veins. There are some critics who would say it is not. It is true that – in theory – the pressure applied when rolling the calf, for example, could damage the tissue and cause an existing blood clot to come loose. According to this logic, however, the best course of action for people with weakened veins would be to stay in bed all day where no harm can come to them – which, of course, makes no sense at all.

In the long term, it has also been shown that certain ways of applying pressure, be it with compression stockings or hydrotherapy, can actually strengthen the veins. It all comes down to applying the right amount of pressure. And as with anything else, sometimes people will take an approach to such an extreme that they cause themselves harm. This can even happen with basic activities like drinking water, hiking or swimming. The important question is therefore how likely the individual is to use the method in an unhelpful way, and how often injury occurs. In rugby, for instance, the likelihood of injury is one in every 40 hours played; for Nordic walking, it is one in every thousand hours.

As yet, there are no reliable statistics concerning this matter for roller treatment. From my own observation of the huge pool of people who use this technique, the risk seems to me to be just as low as with Nordic walking or hiking. I therefore think it would be overkill to suggest that no one should be using foam rollers without expert guidance. The only exception is people with weak veins who, as I have already mentioned, should definitely seek advice from a medical specialist before considering using this technique. For everybody else, I would say to approach the roller with as much enthusiasm but also as much caution as you would new walking poles or when starting a new fitness regime.

Model	Application	Tool
Regular roller	▶ Suitable for most uses	
Very soft roller	▶ Unbeatable as an entry-level model for many users ▶ Allows for gentle rolling of sensitive body parts	
Very hard roller	▶ Initially, this roller should only be used by individuals or for body parts that are particularly strong and robust ▶ Suitable for gradually increasing the intensity of the practice as the body becomes more resilient following several months of regular rolling treatment	
Peanut-shaped roller	▶ Ideal for treating the spine, especially in individuals with particularly prominent spinous processes	
Air-filled roller	▶ Even distribution of pressure across the surface of the body improves the 'sponge effect' (rehydration)	
Textured roller	▶ More intense stimulation (metabolic stimulation) of individual areas. If you keep rolling repeatedly, eventually all the areas you treat will be subjected to this more intense level of stimulation ▶ Individuals with particularly soft connective tissue should exercise caution if using this roller	
Ribbed roller	▶ Similar effect to the textured roller ▶ Can also achieve a localised sponge effect, by pressing out the tissue in the rolling direction; this is particularly good for chronic swelling	

Model	Application	Tool
Ball roller	► Targeted treatment of individual pressure points ► If you lay on your stomach and prop up your upper body, this can also be good for treating the area around the shoulders and chest muscles on the front of the body	
Double ball	► Good for the neck and spine; similar to peanut-shaped rollers ► As long as the distance between the two balls corresponds to the position of the back muscles, a double ball can be more suitable for back massage than a roller	
Rod roller	► Often gives the user more control of the roller and how they apply it to their own body, such as: back massage in a seated position or with one leg laid over the rod	
Heated roller or ball	► When applied for several minutes at a time, these can be highly effective at relaxing particularly knotted areas	
Vibrating ball, wand or roller – high vibration	► Increased metabolic activation and proprioceptive stimulation ► Often accelerates regeneration in individuals with muscle soreness	
Vibrating ball, wand or roller – low vibration	► Improves body awareness ► Ideal for extra relaxation – before sleep, for example	

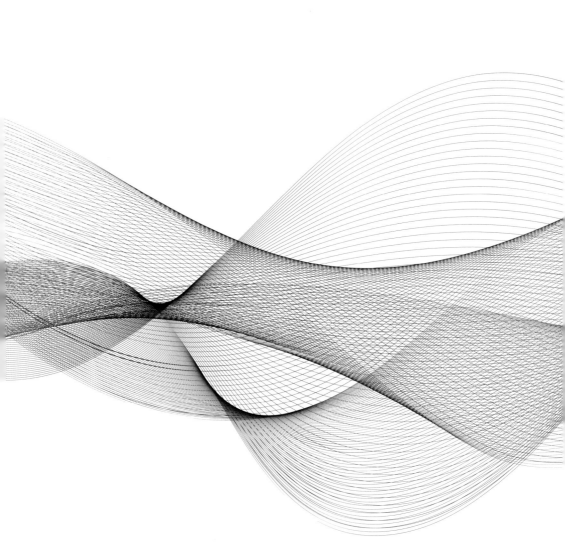

Chapter 5

Fascial fitness: healthy eating and lifestyle

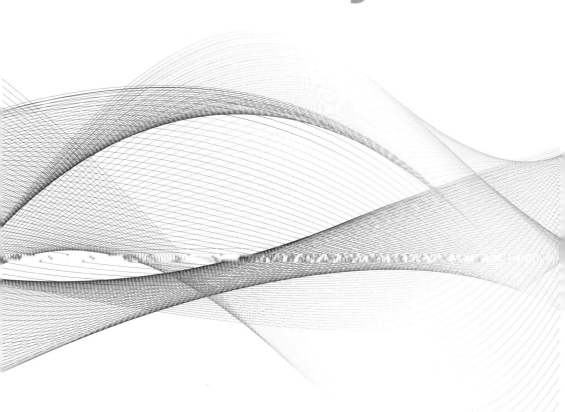

This short chapter is dedicated to the subject of diet and lifestyle. In our line of work, people often ask us questions like: What should we be eating? How does nutrition affect fascia? Which minerals, micronutrients or vitamins are best for fascia?

Generally speaking, it's pretty obvious: to keep our fascia fit or restore its fitness, we need to be leading a healthy lifestyle. This is almost self-evident, as ultimately the maintenance of the whole body depends on us eating nutritious food and getting plenty of sleep. Most of the advice in this area is already very well known and self-explanatory, so there's no need for us to list it all for you here. However, there are a few factors you can focus on and a few tweaks you could make here and there to give your connective tissue the chance to thrive.

Our tips are based on well-founded nutritional and health guidelines. However, this is not comprehensive nutrition advice. We simply wish to highlight the things that are especially important for fascia. At the end, I will give you a few tips that I personally find helpful.

Maintaining a healthy weight

Try to avoid being overweight, as carrying too much weight puts excess pressure on the subsystems of the bones, joints, ligaments, tendons and fascia. In addition, you may suffer from greatly reduced mobility. By 'overweight', we mainly mean storing too much fat in the adipose tissue, which is in fact part of the connective tissue. When the cells in this tissue are congested, they produce unhelpful hormones and neurotransmitters that trigger a constant state of mild inflammation in the whole body. This is proven to be damaging to your metabolism, especially in fascia. We also can't ignore that there is a cosmetic element to being overweight: nowadays, visible cellulite on the stomach, legs, buttocks and underarms can significantly affect how we feel about ourselves and our general sense of well-being.

No smoking!

Smoking damages the entire body, and if you really want to improve the health of your fascia, then you should not smoke at all. Smoking hugely increases the number of free radicals in the body, which damage the cells and cause the oxygen content of the blood to fall. In addition, the inhalation of nicotine poisons the blood vessels, constricting them and causing stress. The end result is that fascia receives fewer nutrients. Evidence shows that smokers are much more susceptible to back pain, cartilage injury, arthritis and slipped discs. All of these disorders are associated with insufficient nutrient and blood supply to the connective tissue and fascia.

Staying hydrated

Because the connective tissue contains up to 70 percent water, it needs plenty of it to stay healthy. Try to drink between 1 and 1.5 litres of water a day – and that does mean water – not juice, lemonade, cola, milk-based drinks or coffee. These are all stimulants, and not reliable for quenching thirst. It's best if you can get used to drinking normal tap water rather than sparkling water, as you can get it anywhere and it's usually good quality. Performance athletes may find they need more than the recommended amount; drink as much as you need. However, drinking massive amounts of water is not recommended. In fact, there have been extreme cases where people have died from drinking too much water. Equally, don't be under any illusions – drinking water alone will not cure the brittleness in your lumbar fascia or replenish the fluid in your Achilles tendon. That is because the fluid absorption in fascia is not linked to the gastrointestinal tract. The fluid

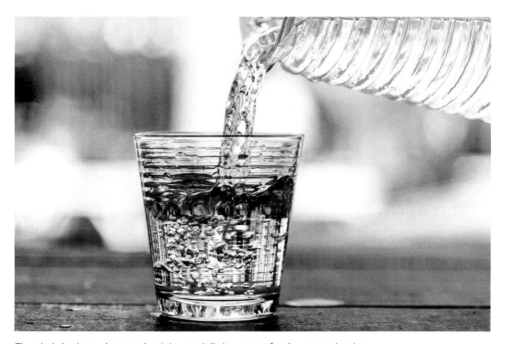

The whole body needs water, but it is especially important for the connective tissue.

only replenishes itself when the tissue is squeezed out like a sponge. This is due to the specific water-binding process inside fascia. When the sponge – i.e. the tissue – is not squeezed regularly enough, it is unable to absorb the new, fresh water that it needs, no matter how much of the stuff you gulp down each day. The key is to make your tissue thirsty by making it work – ideally using the exercises described in our program.

Getting enough protein

Protein fibres are the most important basic material in fascia. In order to produce these fibres, the body itself needs protein – and specifically that which contains certain amino acids. It cannot produce these amino acids itself so it has to take this protein from our food. For the production of connective tissue cell fibres, an adequate intake of protein is therefore essential. Animal protein is better for this than plant protein, as it contains more amino acids. It's therefore best to eat plenty of high-quality meat and free-range eggs, as well as fish, cheese and other dairy products. For those who follow a vegetarian diet, it is particularly important to make sure you're getting enough protein from lentils, beans or other legumes, as well as eggs and dairy products. It is wise to familiarise yourself with good

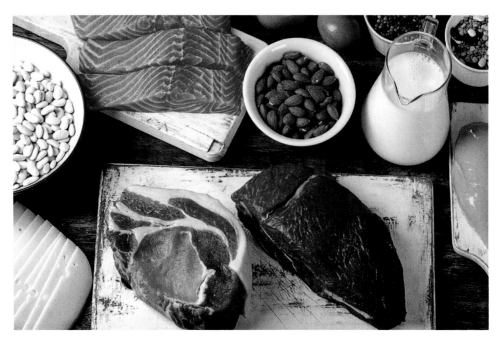

Meat and dairy products provide particularly high amounts of valuable protein. Vegetarians can get theirs from eggs and legumes.

recipe books and scientific nutrient tables regarding the right sources of protein.

Vitamin C for collagen

Collagen synthesis in the connective tissue depends on us having enough vitamin C – it acts as a kind of glue that the cells use to hold all the fibres together. If there is a significant deficit of vitamin C in the body, this leads of symptoms of deficiency in the tissue because it interrupts collagen synthesis. Symptoms include bleeding gums, poor wound healing, peeling of the periosteum, and cornification – all of which are symptoms of the deficiency disease known as scurvy. Vitamin C is therefore very important for the connective tissue. A genuine deficiency is quite rare, but do pay attention to whether or not you are getting enough vitamin C; and don't be deceived into thinking that fruit is the best source of vitamin C. For example, there is very little vitamin C in apples, and even the amount found in lemons and oranges is less than in many locally sourced vegetables. Have a look at a vitamin table and you will see that certain members of the cabbage family such as broccoli, cauliflower, kale, white cabbage and savoy, all contain more vitamin C than citrus fruits. Other vegetables that are packed with vitamin C include spinach, fennel, parsley, chillies and especially peppers. In fact, even potatoes and chips

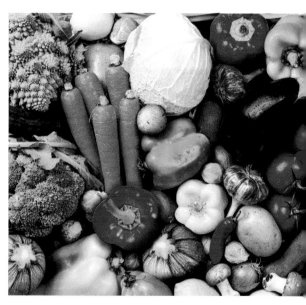

The vegetables most rich in vitamin C include various types of cabbage and peppers.

are reliable sources of vitamin C. In the summer, strawberries and native berries also make excellent local sources. Tropical fruits like kiwi, guava and papaya are also rich in vitamin C, as are acerola cherries, which usually come processed in juice or powder form. However, eating plenty of fresh vegetables is the most convenient and economical way of getting enough vitamin C, and they are better for your metabolism.

Zinc, copper, magnesium and potassium for fitness

Zinc is an essential trace element that is involved in protein, fat, and cell metabolism;

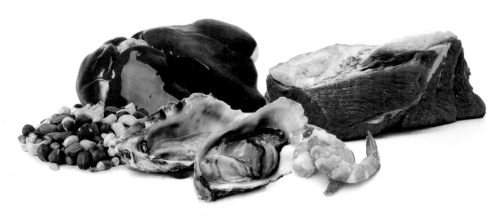

Liver, oysters and prawns are particularly rich in zinc, as are nuts and meat.

it strengthens the immune system and affects insulin production. It is essential for many hormonal functions, including thyroid hormones and testosterone production. Testosterone ensures solid connective tissue in both men and women. Zinc also plays a role in wound healing, and is contained in the walls of connective tissue cells as well as being productive in the synthesis of collagen. A lack of zinc manifests itself through impaired wound healing, weak connective tissue and general susceptibility to infection. Good sources of zinc are beef and pork, eggs, milk, cheese, legumes, nuts, seafood and offal. Zinc is absorbed more efficiently from meat and animal products than from vegetables.

Only recently, studies have shown that another trace element of particular benefit to fascia health is copper. When the body produces new collagen through healthy stimulation of fascia, something called enzymatic crosslinks are also created. Their role is to connect adjacent collagen and elastin fibres to one another. These crosslinks increase the tissue's resistance to injury and are generally seen as a positive phenomenon. Copper is an essential building block that the body needs to manufacture these links, but it cannot produce it by itself. Copper is found mainly in fish, nuts, legumes, seeds, cocoa, and in offal such as the liver.

Magnesium and potassium also affect cell metabolism and growth, collagen synthesis and water levels; their intake should be adequately monitored. Good sources of magnesium are mineral water, many nuts and particularly sunflower seeds. Mushrooms, bananas, beans, cheese, spinach and potatoes are high in potassium.

Getting enough sleep

When we sleep, our entire system, but in particular the connective tissues and the intervertebral discs, undergoes a process of regeneration. Provided that they are rested for long enough, the intervertebral discs can absorb liquid again, meaning they are able to obtain fresh nutrients. In addition, only in deep sleep is the growth hormone HGH secreted, which stimulates the synthesis of collagen in the connective tissue cells. Adequate and restful sleep are therefore extremely important. Here are some tips for good sleep hygiene: Go to bed at a similar time every night and try not to stay up past the natural point of tiredness. Get enough sleep. For most people, this means between seven and nine hours. Take breaks during the day, especially at lunchtime. Physiologically, the body is programed to rest at midday, and not to speed up. The more you adhere to this rhythm, the less stress you will put on your body. Your fascia will thank you.

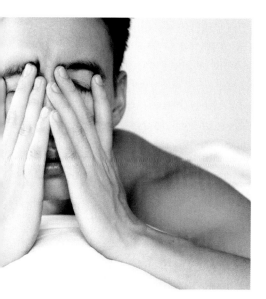

Lack of sleep also causes stress in the connective tissue.

From silica to gelatine – what supplements should we be taking?

Silica, silicon, vitamin C, zinc, minerals, trace elements and vitamin B complex are all recommended for the connective tissues. You can simply take a pill, instead of painstakingly preparing food that contains the perfect balance of all these vitamins and minerals. That said, it is indisputable that vitamins and trace elements are more effective if they enter the body in the form of real food, because food is also full of other healthy materials. Foods naturally rich in vitamins include roughage, specifically vegetables and fruit, which contain many more secondary plant substances than just vitamins and trace elements. Likewise, meat, eggs and milk provide essential fats and amino acids. These ensure that the vitamins can be properly absorbed by the body.

Zinc is a definite exception. It is one of the few trace elements in which there can be a latent deficiency, so you couldn't go far wrong with a short course of zinc tablets every now and then. Nonetheless, it is wise to seek advice from a pharmacist or a doctor. B vitamins, of which there are eight in total, belong to the group of vitamins that it is helpful to replenish now and again, especially after infectious diseases, periods of stress, or when following a vegetarian diet. They are stored in the body, but the reserves can dwindle, especially during periods of unusually high stress. To top up the storage, it is recommendable to take a vitamin B complex, but once again it is wise to seek advice from your doctor or pharmacist.

Silica is a mixture of substances, one of which is silicon. Traditionally, it is considered in alternative therapy circles to be most useful for connective tissue, hair and nails. Actually, silicon is a component of connective tissue. Whether silica, when taken as a supplement, has the desired effect in terms of fascia regeneration, is yet to be proved. Some years ago, silica products came into disrepute having been found to be contaminated and contain sand, as well as being linked to kidney damage. The Consumer Council of Hamburg issued a damning verdict after federal and state authorities examined silica products, and doctors assertively advised against using them.

It is another matter when it comes to gelatine, with the latest research confirming that this animal protein can help build the connective tissue that contains collagen. This had been the assumption for many years, as it was well known that taking gelatine helps promote wound healing and support intensive athletic performance training. Gelatine is an ingredient in many foods, such as gummy bears and jelly, which is probably why we don't really see it as a medicinal or dietary supplement. Yet, as far back as the Middle Ages, the German Abbess and healer Hildegard von Bingen recommended a broth made from boiled calves' feet to soothe aching muscles, which would have been full of naturally dissolved gelatine. The main reason this was so effective is that the collagen from the bones and connective tissue of the animals was boiled for such a long time that the heat would dissolve the rope-like arrangement of the fibres, leaving behind the essential components. These are the building blocks of protein, which help the body to produce collagen. This is backed up by science, with several major studies having shown that regular consumption of gelatine, plus plenty of exercise, increases collagen synthesis in fascia. In one of the studies, adults who were given several grams of gelatine powder on a daily basis performed better in a rope skipping exercise – in terms of their jumping performance – than the control

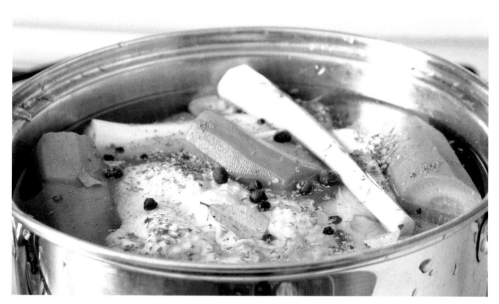

Granny's chicken soup is making a comeback: we now have a scientific explanation for its anti-inflammatory effects.

group who received a placebo. Anti-inflammatory effects have also been documented in association with the specific components of collagen, known as 'peptides', which come from gelatine. They are already being used to treat various ailments, including arthritis of the joints. In fact, it may well be the case that these specific collagen peptides are absorbed even more effectively by the body than normal gelatine. Further research is needed to confirm this.

If you want to consume gelatine, you can buy it in purified form as a powder or capsules from chemists, pharmacies and online. It is usually derived from the subcutaneous connective tissue in pork or beef. You can also buy fish gelatine, but there is no vegetarian alternative. Fish gelatine can also be bought either online or from pharmacies, but it is much more expensive than beef or pork gelatine. There is no purely vegetarian variant because the main component has to be collagen, which is an animal protein.

Incidentally, gelatine also reveals why Granny's chicken soup has such magical healing powers. In folk medicine, chicken broth has been recommended for centuries as a cure for colds. As recent studies have shown, its remedial effects seem to be largely down to the anti-inflammatory properties of the dissolved collagen components. As with Hilde's calves' foot broth, heat is also key. For a really good broth, the chicken bones should be boiled over a low heat for as long as possible – at least an hour.

The great sugar debate

Sugar has become the source of much controversy. Anti-sugar activists are calling it a deadly poison, while the sweet-toothed among us cling to our little treats for dear life, the level-headed warn against black-and-white thinking, and the industry is doing everything it can to avoid a drop in sales. However, this book is not designed to provide general nutritional advice, but to offer advice on what nourishes fascia or what might damage it. One thing is for sure: too much of anything is always unhealthy. The same goes for sugar, which is ultimately a luxury food that our bodies do not really need.

That said, there is little proof of the many evils that sugar has been claimed to have in relation to connective tissue in recent years. Some researchers have warned that sugar is deposited in the fascia from the blood, causing the tissue to yellow and stiffen. As evidence of this, they presented impressive tissue samples from the fascia of young, healthy people in comparison with that of certain patients.

However, this phenomenon is not caused by sugar as an ingredient of our food. It is a result of the interaction between various different types of sugar found in the blood – especially fructose, but also glucose and others – with protein. The reasons behind this are increased levels of blood sugar and type 2 diabetes. Many people now suffer from this as our modern-day lifestyles often send our blood sugar regulation out of whack. The factors at play here are too little exercise, stress, lack of sleep and genetic predisposition, as well as consuming too many calories, binge eating and carrying excess weight. However, the problem is not caused specifically by household sugar. Even those who do not eat many sugary foods can have type 2 diabetes and high blood sugar. The common factor, however, is that they overeat. In fact, being overweight is the biggest risk factor for high blood sugar. We have already touched upon this, and the advice we can offer on the matter is really quite general. Eating sensibly, maintaining healthy blood sugar levels and avoiding carrying excess weight has a variety of benefits for your connective tissue. That's why we would suggest having regular check-ups with your doctor. If you already suffer from high blood sugar levels, insulin resistance, type 2 diabetes or a lipid metabolism disorder, you may be storing increased levels of modified sugar crystals in your connective tissue. It is therefore very important that you follow the advice of your doctor and a qualified dietician.

Inflammation and fascia

For those who suffer from chronic illnesses and complaints, as well as unexplained pain, the recurring factor tends to be inflammation in the body. Doctors now know that inflammatory processes are the number one cause of the dreaded atherosclerosis or 'hardening of the arteries', which in turn leads to heart attacks. Many other diseases, such as type 2 diabetes and certain forms of rheumatism, including arthritis, are also caused by chronic inflammation – as is asthma and, in some cases, even depression and Alzheimer's disease. However, there are no firm conclusions as to what causes this inflammation, whether or not it can really be controlled with the right diet and lifestyle choices, as many claim, and why certain people appear to be genetically predisposed to inflammation – within the blood vessels, for example. In recent years, there has been more and more focus on silent or hidden inflammation.

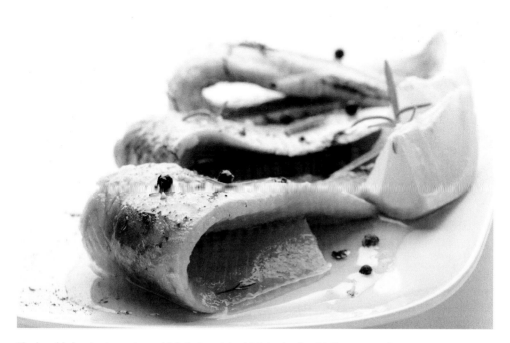

The humble herring is one type of fish that contains high levels of anti-inflammatory fats.

This occurs throughout the entire body, putting constant strain on the immune system and is considered a common factor in poor health. Possible triggers include undiscovered inflammation in the dental root and chronic cystitis. In some cases, inflammation may be found in the blood, with no identifiable cause whatsoever. A high level of pro-inflammatory molecules in the blood has a negative effect on collagen synthesis and therefore damage the fascia. Inflammatory swelling can also develop during exercise and persist for several days or longer. To find out whether you have hidden inflammation, you can ask your doctor to do a simple blood test (CRP test).

What is certain is that getting enough sleep, avoiding stress and following a few basic dietary rules can arm the body against inflammation. For people who suffer from inflammatory forms of rheumatism or gout, it is of course particularly important that you follow the advice of your doctor and/or dietician. For those in good health and athletes who may be aware of some of the dietary factors that promote or prevent inflammation, here are a few basic rules: Yes, it's good to eat

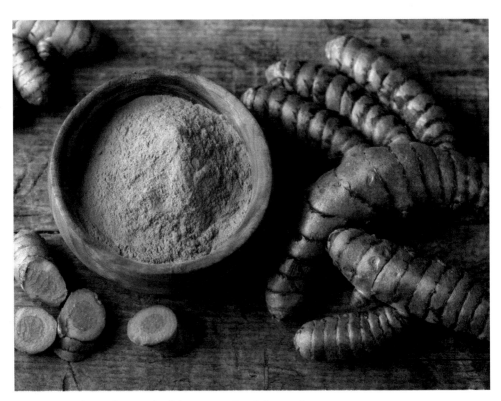

Turmeric contains a substance that is known to reduce inflammation.

oily fish like salmon, mackerel or herring, ideally twice a week. That's because they contain omega-3 fatty acids, which have been shown to have anti-inflammatory effects. Important fatty acids can also be found in certain plant-based products, such as linseed oil and walnuts. And yes, getting enough fibre from vegetables and whole grains is a good idea, as is eating yogurt and fermented milk products, which promote healthy intestinal flora. The more you feed your gut bacteria with the right kinds of fibre, the better your intestinal flora will be and the stronger your immune system. Chronic inflammation overwhelms the immune system, but nurturing a healthy intestinal flora can help it to recover. All of these things help fight inflammation. Ultimately, this puts the body in a better position to heal any injuries in the fascia and to keep the connective tissue in good working order. Suggestions for finding general information about nutrition and inflammation can be found in the further reading section.

Tips from me to you

I like to make my own little remedy using certain herbal extracts, vitamins and minerals. It's not something I take all the time; I take breaks in between. The ingredients that I tend to use include zinc, vitamin C, copper, powdered gelatine or collagen peptides, as well as curcumin and green tea powder. Curcumin is the main ingredient of the Indian spice turmeric and is used as a folk remedy in Ayurvedic medicine. Modern research has certified that this bright yellow spice does genuinely have anti-inflammatory properties. Curcumin also has an impact on the growth of certain tumours. The important thing to keep in mind is that the body absorbs this active ingredient much better if the curcumin is administered along with a little pepper. The capsules and other preparations available in shops therefore often contain a mixture of curcumin and pepper.

If you take turmeric powder yourself, add some freshly ground black pepper to it. You could also try the classic recipe for 'golden milk' – a warm, spicy milk drink made with turmeric and black pepper. Similar beneficial effects can be derived from green tea or green tea powder. The active ingredients in green tea leaves reduce the number of free radicals in the body and are therefore considered to prevent and reduce inflammation in several ways. During the day, I occasionally treat myself to the particularly highly concentrated variant, matcha tea, which is the kind used in Japanese tea ceremony. Matcha is green tea ground into a powder.

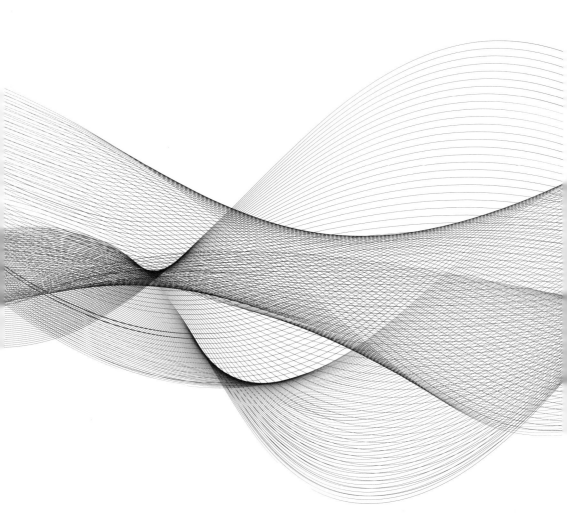

Chapter 6

Periodised fascia training for speed, power and injury resilience

Bill Parisi & Johnathon Allen

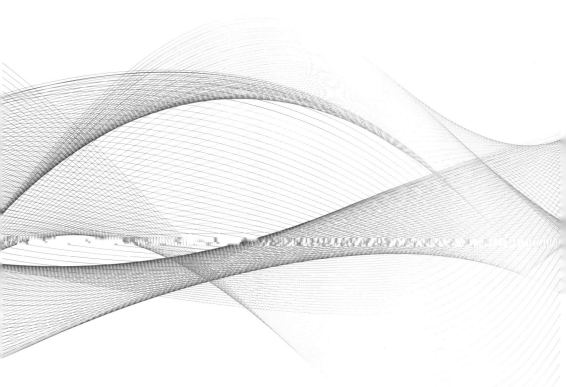

In the 1990s, the common assumption was that speed was not something you could dramatically improve through training. It was a genetic gift. You were either born to be fast or you weren't. It was believed that if you had more fast-twitch Type II muscle fibres and a leaner frame, you were inevitably going to be faster. While there's obviously some inherent truth to that perception (looking at you, Usain Bolt), it turns out that this is not the end of the story. But, hey, we were also logging onto the Internet with dial-up modems and calling that fast. And, just like the Internet, our technology, research and understanding of speed have evolved significantly over the past few decades to give us new insights. Not only have we proven that human speed can be significantly enhanced through targeted training, we have a much better understanding of how and why (Clark and Weyand, 2014).

In addition to demonstrating that the fascial system is both adaptable and trainable, modern research and imaging technology suggest it may play a significant role in the body's ability to generate speed in all of its many forms (Schleip and Müller, 2013) – from running a sub-10-second 100-metre dash, to throwing a 100 mph fast ball, and delivering a lightning-fast knockout punch. In all these examples, speed comes from multiple anatomical systems working together in a highly coordinated unison, enabled by the body's integrated myofascial web. Of course, when I first began developing speed training programs there was not a lot of hard science available to explain how the fascia system was involved. I just knew that what we were doing worked. In fact, over the past 30-plus years, the Parisi Training System has produced first-round draft picks in every professional sport – including more than 145 NFL draft picks – and a host of Olympic medallists and champion UFC fighters. I originally learned many of the techniques used to achieve these results when I travelled to Finland, after graduating from High School, to train with the top javelin throwers and coaches in the world. As a short, stocky Italian, I'm not genetically designed for throwing aluminium spears long distances, so I needed all the help I could get. This desire to be great at something I wasn't naturally gifted at sent me on a lifelong quest to learn from the best.

While I was in Finland, I was exposed to advanced functional training and medicine ball techniques I hadn't previously seen in the US – techniques that I now understand optimise the adaptive remodelling and elastic properties of the fascia system. This functional approach to three-dimensional, fascia-focused training allowed me to rise to the top of American collegiate competition and get my education paid for by becoming one of the best NCAA Division I javelin throwers in the nation, and the all-time record holder at Iona College. In the process, I learned that throwing things is one of the most complete forms of athleticism there is. To be a great thrower, you need powerful legs and a stiff, super-strong core. You also need the ability to harness the elastic storage properties of your tendons and fascia system to channel tremendous amounts of force from your lower body through your trunk, torso, shoulder, arm, elbow, wrist and fingers. It is a whole-body experience (Naito et al, 2011). There is a reason many books about fascia have had javelin throwers on the cover.

This is where I feel it is important to pause for a moment and point out that there are a lot of very smart researchers and practitioners in this book who know significantly more than I do about the science of fascia. I'm not a scientist. I'm an aggregator of knowledge and experience. I'm a coach who wants to get the best out of his athletes. And I'm certainly not the smartest guy in the room. What I've found is that you don't need to be the smartest guy in the room if you can identify who the smart people are and learn from them. That said, we all have our own unique backgrounds, histories, and specialties – just like fascia tissue – and we all have something to contribute. So, I strongly encourage you to read the cutting-edge information in this book with a hungry, open mind and apply whatever principles you learn from it to your practice in your own way so you can bring something uniquely 'you' to it. Find the top experts and learn from them. Look at what the research tells you. Allow yourself to be surprised by the results. And then evolve your approach in response, because this is new territory, and one of the most important things that I've learned over the past few years while exploring this subject is that fascia loves variability – variability in load, variability in movement and variability of vectors (Zügel et al, 2018). This is why basketball players tend to be inherently fascia-driven athletes. The sport of basketball is a three-dimensional game with constantly changing variables happening on multiple planes with submaximal loads and explosive movements that engage the entire body from foot to finger in a bullet-fast chain reaction of proprioception and elasticity. Spend three-plus hours a day playing basketball from a very young age (and avoid injury) and you will likely develop thicker Achilles tendons with powerful dynamic recoil properties that give you kangaroo-like abilities for jumping, accelerating and rapidly changing direction (Wiesinger et al, 2017). This was the original *aha!* moment that drove me to become obsessed with the subject of fascia in the first place: I was watching my son, Will, compete alongside 15- and 16-year-old kids with outstanding athleticism as he toured the country playing in the Nike AAU basketball tournament. Many of these teens were playing above the rim and crossing the floor in five or six strides, but they spent little, if any, time traditionally training in the gym. They didn't do anatomically-targeted strength workouts like "chest day" or "leg day." They didn't do periodised training. They just played a lot of basketball. That was when I realised there was something deeper going on and began my quest to understand the science behind it. I read every research paper I could find. I grabbed my writer sidekick, Johnathon Allen, and set out on a year-long road trip to interview every expert on the subject who would talk to us so we could write a book about it. In the process, I discovered that this mysterious "something" was the fascia system and that these kids were naturally training and tuning its powerful elastic amplification properties simply by playing basketball all day. The question this realisation led me to, as a strength and conditioning coach, was: How do we create a fascia-aware curriculum backed by the latest research that any athlete or coach can use to improve athletic performance and injury resilience?

Fascia training 101

I like to keep things simple, so let's start with the basics. According to Davis's Law, fascial tissue continuously remodels itself in triple-helix strands of collagen produced by thousands of tiny fibroblast cells that organise along the lines of load and stress in the body's extra-cellular matrix using a biological process called mechanotransduction (Ingber, 1998). That's a lot of big scientific words that essentially mean the net of your body-wide fascia system is constantly remodelling itself based on your movements, loading patterns, diet and lifestyle – just like a plant. If you sit hunched over at a desk all day, you will probably develop densely matted concentrations of collagen in the myofascial layers of your shoulders and your upper and lower back where the stress and load are concentrated. Without a regular program of variable movements that activate those tissues and pump viscous fluid into them, they will eventually harden into dense adhesions that limit your mobility. On the other hand, if you spend your days working on a farm or an Alaskan tuna boat struggling against gravity under constantly variable loads happening on multiple planes that challenge your body's kinetic chain in frequently awkward positions (and avoid injury), you will develop a resilient three-dimensional fascia system and thick, powerful tendons that can give you the ability to generate tremendous amounts of force, despite having a leaner/smaller frame than someone who bulks up at the gym. Science is showing us that this enhanced capability for power generation comes from the elastic amplification properties of tendons and fascia tissue, and a neurological chain reaction of co-contractions happening across multiple myofascial structures that combine to create a finely-tuned balance of stability and mobility (Maas & Sandercock, 2010). If you doubt this assertion, challenge a farm kid or deep-sea fisherman to a wrestling match and see how it goes. Actually, you should definitely not do that. But this takes us back to the million-dollar question: How do we harness this biological dynamic to create functional athletic training programs that improve speed, power and injury resilience?

Fascial tissue and its behaviour are based on its biological structure. If we understand the basic structure of fascia and how it behaves, we can understand how to train it. Observed simply, fascia is made up of cells, fibres, the extra cellular matrix and water. When it comes to the cells within fascia, we have fibroblasts, mast cells, adipose cells and macrophages, and all of them do very specific things. During the tissue remodelling phase of healing, macrophage activity and collagenase enzymes clean up the old tissue so we can lay down the new. Fibroblasts are the cells that lay down the new. Fibroblasts build fascia just like osteoblasts build bone. They line up along the lines of stress – or 'load paths' – and produce the protein

fibres of collagen, elastin and reticulin. Since farm kids and deep-sea fishermen stress their bodies in all sorts of different lengths, angles and positions, they end up laying down an omnidirectional latticework of protein fibres throughout their bodies that is driven by the wide variety of loading patterns happening along the many different lines of stress they are subjected to.

Importantly, though, fascia tissue remodelling is rate/load specific (Bohm et al, 2014). Elastic energy is stored and released by tendons and fascia tissue very quickly – in less than 1.2 seconds (Kawakam et al, 2002). If a force lasts longer than that, the plasticity properties of fascia will adjust to accommodate the load. This means that training tendons and fascia tissue for more elastic explosiveness requires short, cyclic, quickly repeated motions, such as bouncing, jumping rope, or running on the balls of your feet (as opposed to slower-contraction cycles, such as bicycling or rowing). Another key aspect in this dynamic is that the Type I collagen fibres that store and release elastic energy need to be connected and glued down in the extracellular matrix. They are glued down by a fluid called ground substance, which contains soluble carbohydrate polymers. These polymers take the protein fibres and glue them together omnidirectionally. The other critical element in fascia tissue is water. We have either bound water or unbound water in our tissues. Unbound water consists of free-floating H_2O molecules that are not bonded with each other. Bound water is where H_2O molecules are bonded with each other, and a hydrophilic surface, in their vicinity. When that happens, there is strong evidence to suggest that fascia becomes stiffer and more dynamic because it is more resistant to compression (Pollack, 2001). If you are an athlete and you have stiffer, more dynamic fascia tissue, that means you are wearing a kind of internal weightlifting compression suit that is both tighter and more-stretchy. Which is a win/win. This means we want the water in fascia to be bound. This can be achieved through specific movement techniques, stretching, foam rolling, mechanical manipulation, eating fresh food and drinking plenty of water, alongside other strategies.

Vector variability

One of the first things to explore when designing a periodised training program is anatomical adaptation and the importance of vector variability in preparing the body for increased levels of exertion. The basic periodisation premise is that the preparation phase of anatomical adaptation leads to strength, which leads to power (i.e. the expression of strength), which leads to speed, agility and quickness. Traditionally, weight, rep schemes, tempos and rest periods were the only variables in the anatomical adaptation phase of a periodised training program. Typically, weights would be used to do mostly linear, sagittal-plane movements in the gym, with higher reps for anatomical adaptation, lower reps with heavier weights for strength, and even lower reps using lighter weights and faster bar movements for power. However, with a fascia-aware approach to periodisation, the process of anatomical adaptation is not just a matter of repeating the same movement patterns over and over with the same tempos along the same lines of stress. A fascia-aware approach to anatomical adaptation should include a variety of loads, vectors and angles, which stimulate omnidirectional tissue remodelling from the outset. This is because fibroblasts will lay down collagen in a more balanced latticework of fibres that provides increased shape stability, greater elastic recoil capability and more resistance to deformation which helps improve injury resilience. If tissues in the ankles, knees, hip, trunk, arms and shoulders are exposed to different loads at different angles during the anatomical adaptation phase, the power of omnidirectional tissue remodelling can be harnessed across the entire body. This makes vector variability a key ingredient in anatomical adaptation.

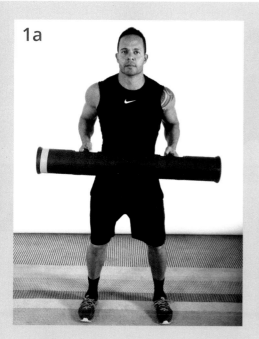

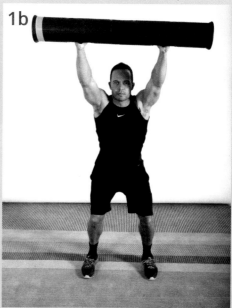

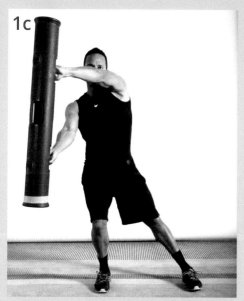

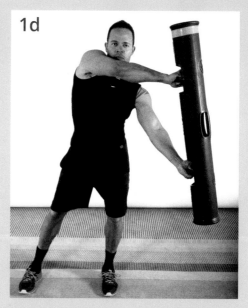

1a – 1d: The Box Pattern drill provides vector variability. It activates the core and fascia connections in a whole-body chain reaction along the frontal plane. Work with any loaded movement tool such as a ViPR PRO (pictured), medicine ball, or kettlebell to achieve vector variability using the external load and gravity as drivers. 1. Start by holding the load in an athletic stance. 2. Raise the load overhead. 3. Rotate the load vertically while lunging to the right. 4. Return to the overhead position. 5. Rotate the load vertically while lunging to the left. 6. Repeat an equal number of reps on each side (6–8).

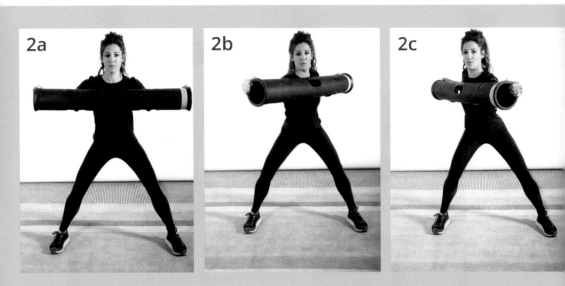

2a – 2c: *The Alternate Interior Reach drill is another example of vector variability. It activates the core and engages fascia connections in a chain reaction along the transverse plane. 1. Start by holding the load by the outside edges in an athletic stance. 2. Rotate torso while reaching across the frontal plane as far as possible with each hand. 4. Repeat an equal number of reps on each side (6–8).*

Odd position strength

For the strength training phase of a fascia-aware periodisation program, we want to focus on working with submaximal loads in odd positions at length. The idea with this approach is to load odd positions at length so we can engage tissue paths across the entire body over multiple joints on all three planes. To be clear, we're not saying that shortening under load is bad and lengthening under load is good. We're saying that they're both good – they are just different inputs that get different results. The issue is that we have done one of them in the training and conditioning world forever, which is doing link-actions over joints where the muscles shorten, and one or two levers close a joint angle. However, what we aim to achieve from a fascia-training perspective is to subject the body to a variety of different load paths on all three planes in a way that involves multiple joints, tissues and structures. This allows us to develop better shape stability and strength across the entire fabric of the body, not just over a local joint or segment.

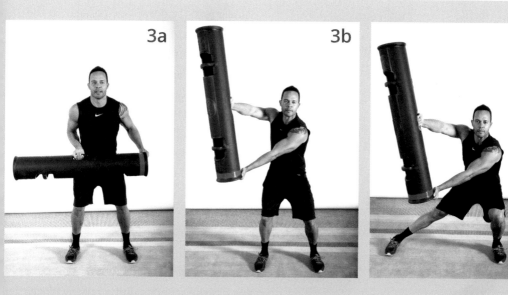

3a – 3c: *The Flag Lunge helps develop odd-position strength by activating whole-body load paths and co-contractions in three dimensions on all three planes. Work with any loaded movement tool such as a ViPR PRO (pictured), medicine ball, or kettle bell to develop odd-position strength using the external load and gravity as drivers. 1. Start by holding a load at midline with a shovel grip in an athletic stance. 2. Raise the load laterally to one side, like a flag. 3. Lunge across the frontal plane in the opposite direction of the load while exhaling forcefully. 4. Return to the starting position. 5. Repeat an equal number of repetitions on each side (6–8).*

Power and speed

In the world of athletic training, power is considered an expression of strength. If strength is being expressed at speed, it is often described in the industry as either speed strength or strength-speed. While these terms are sometimes used interchangeably, they involve different training approaches and outcomes. Speed-strength refers to moving a load at a high rate of speed (e.g. a lineman in football pushing his opponent), while strength-speed refers to moving a relatively heavy load with the intention of moving it as fast as possible (e.g. Olympic lifting). In the power development phase of periodised training, the focus should be on movements that involve rapid oscillating speeds and rebound motions where the contact times are under 1.2 seconds (Kawakami et al, 2002). This means doing things such as bouncing a medicine ball against a wall, jumping rope, running on the balls of the feet, or quickly moving a submaximal load overhead from one shoulder to the other. When these inputs are done at a faster athletic pace, they will stimulate cell

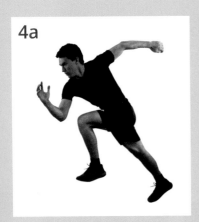

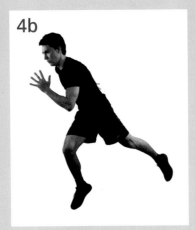

4a – 4b: Power Bounds develop the ability to use the "catapult effect" of the tendons and fascia system. Powerful extension and flexion from the ankle, knee, hip, core and shoulder are needed to maximise force generation. This exercise forces the tendons and fascia system to engage in the high-intensity movement of loaded single-leg bounding. Step 1: Begin in a sprinter's stance and start by exploding backward off one leg while driving the opposite knee forward and the opposite arm backward. Step 2: Let the ground come to you on each stride. Upon landing, immediately explode off the ground again into the next stride driving the opposite arm and leg backward. Step 3: Repeat the power bounds continuously while striving to cover more horizontal distance on each side. Step 4: Perform for 20–40 yards for 4–8 sets.

signalling to lay down new collagen in the fascia tissue to increase elastic recoil power. The elastic recoil power of collagen fibre is best exemplified by a kangaroo's astounding ability to jump 40 feet at a time in rapid succession and achieve speeds of up to 40 mph. Studies show that this impressive ability does not come from kangaroos having more fast twitch muscle fibres than other animals, as was originally thought (in fact, they have roughly the same amount of Type II muscle fibres as koala bears), it comes from the stored potential energy in the collagen-rich fascia tissue of their massive hindleg tendons and a pulsing elastic recoil dynamic called the "catapult effect" (Kram & Dawson, 1998). Humans are the only primates who have this same biological ability. The catapult effect is enabled by the surrounding muscles, which pre-contract isometrically to stretch the attached connective tissues – loading them like a stretched rubber band – and then quickly relax to release the stored elastic energy in an explosive pulse of force (Kawakami et al, 2002). The key to harnessing this powerful dynamic is the ability to create pulses of "super-stiffness" across the body's integrated myofascial system. Studies conducted by Brown & McGill (2009) revealed that super-stiffness comes from multiple structures co-contracting simultaneously to create a "mechanical composite" of tissues that provide a pulse of rock-solid stability. These pulses of super-stiffness create the anchor points that a kangaroo (or human) needs to rapidly store and release elastic energy relative to the density of collagen fibres in their tendon – like an archer repeatedly firing a compound bow.

Speed, agility and quickness

As a running back in American football, the first line of defence is passed by cutting, darting and quickly changing directions. This rapid darting capability comes from the capacity to convert power into braking and rapid reacceleration in different directions. It requires the ability to instantly read visual and audio cues and quickly respond with appropriate counter-movements while controlling momentum and body mass with pulses of core stiffness. It is a responsive motor skill that is reactive and unplanned. Therefore, it has a significant neurological component that is facilitated in part by the proprioceptive properties of the fascia system (Schleip, 2017). This means power-conversion drills that combine timing, balance and posterior chain strength – like the speed skater bound – are a crucial component in periodised speed training, because they require refined movement literacy, neurological tuning and core strength. Rapid, whole-body compound movements prompt the body to utilise multiple fascial sling systems to absorb force, stabilise momentum, decelerate body mass and produce explosive power

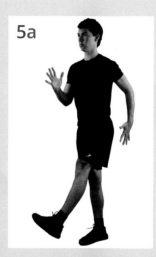

5a

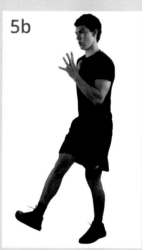

5b

5a – 5b: Straight Leg Bounding is designed to activate the hamstrings and generate horizontal and vertical driving force off the ground. By keeping the leg straight and knees locked it forces the hamstrings to do more of the work as opposed to the quad and glut muscles. Since the hamstrings are complex, two-jointed muscles responsible for hip extension and knee flexion, they are commonly injured. Step 1: Start by standing tall with both legs firmly locked at the knee joint. Step 2: Flex and extend the hip in a shuffle like action while moving forward and slowly increase the intensity of the force production off the ground on each stride. Step 3: Stay leaning slightly forward with a strong active anterior core while syncing the arms with the legs to maximise force production into the ground. Step 4: Do two sets of 20 to 30 yards.

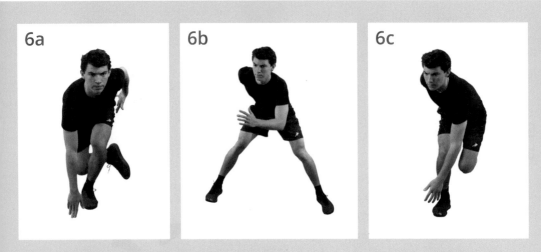

6a – 6c: The speed skater bound is an example of speed-strength conversion. It is a total body movement with a focus on the gluteus maximus and posterior fascia chain. Due to the extreme hip flexion and stretch put on the glute complex while in this bent over position, the initial dynamic contraction challenges the body's fascia slings more than traditional exercises. It is an expression of power and control that relies on neural activity, proprioception and timing. Step 1: Start standing on one leg flexed at the hip and knee with the opposite hand down in front of the grounded leg. Step 2: Dynamically and explosively jump laterally as fast as possible landing and balancing on the opposite leg. Focus on full extension of the hip and knee of the jumping leg while engaging in the lateral movement. Step 3: Immediately upon landing, jump back laterally as fast as possible. Step 4: Repeat continuous jumps for 12–16 total reps, 6–8 reps on each leg for 2–3 sets.

using the catapult effect of the tendons working in conjunction with the myofascial system.

Rest and recovery

When it comes to rest and recovery, the traditional focus is on neural and metabolic recovery periods between workout sessions or circuits. However, there is a strong reason to monitor work-to-rest ratios over the course of each workout, due to the behaviour of the extra cellular matrix. In metabolically-intense Cross-Fit style workouts, injury rates tend to increase after about 30 minutes of exercise (Weisenthal et al, 2014). This is likely to be caused from repetitive, aggressive muscle contractions that push blood and water away from localised areas of the body via muscle pumping and osmotic fluid pressure. When water is pushed out of localised areas, the composition of the extra cellular matrix is changed. The fascia tissue in those areas becomes less dynamic and its stiffness is reduced (Schleip, 2012). However, when water

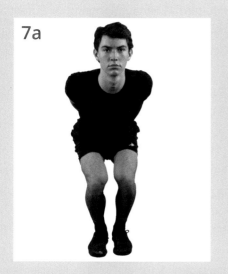 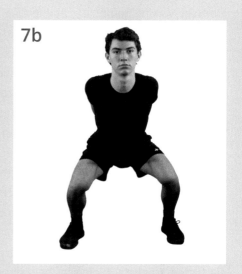

7a – 7b: *Wide-Outs dynamically activate the gluteus medius/maximus and adductor group. By staying low and abducting then, immediately upon ground contact, adducting the legs in a jumping fashion while maintaining balance and a low athletic position, this exercise is a great lateral quickness drill. Step 1: Start in a wide stance squat position with knees in-line with your toes and hands behind your back. Step 2: Without increasing your jump height, bring your feet close together by adducting the legs in a synchronised jump; then land softly maintaining a strong core without increasing the height of your head or hips. Step 3: Immediately upon landing, jump again abducting both legs and separating them back to the starting position. Step 4: Repeat the jumps continuously for two sets of 8 to 12 reps.*

binds to a sugar receptor within the fascia (i.e. it becomes bound water), the tissue becomes stiffer and more resistant to compression. Therefore, it is important to include strategic recovery sessions within workout routines, as opposed to just between sessions. During an intense session, we recommend 10 minutes of rest for every 30 minutes of exhaustive exercise, using restorative pumping-actions that return water and blood to the challenged tissues. This allows water to bind to the fascia cells and sugar receptors to enable a more robust, dynamic and supportive fascial network throughout the workout.

In conclusion, the goal of periodised training is to biologically engineer structural and functional adaptations in the body's tissues over time that improve athletic performance and resiliency. These adaptations are shown to be directly proportional to the mechanical stress inputs created by the intensity (load), volume (quantity), tempo (rate) and frequency of the training. With increasing challenge along omnidirectional paths using varying loads at varying tempos – and enough time to recover and remodel – the fascia tissues will adapt by becoming three-dimensionally stronger and more elastic along the lines of stress. Therefore, a fascia training periodisation program should progress through a series of whole-body exercise routines that emphasise vector variability, then odd-position strength, then power, then speed, agility and quickness – utilising different loads, angles and speeds throughout. By using this structure for a periodised program, the fascia system's natural biological behaviour can be utilised to make athletes stronger, faster and bouncier, with less injury risk – which is the ultimate win.

References

Bohm S, et al, "Human Achilles Tendon Plasticity in Response to Cyclic Strain: Effect of Rate and Duration". J Exp Biol, 2014, Vol 217 (Pt 22), pp 4010–4017.

Brown S H M, McGill, S M, "Transmission of Muscularly Generated Force and Stiffness Between Layers of the Rat Abdominal Wall". Spine, 2009, Vol 34(2), E70–5.

Clark K P, Weyand P G, "Are Running Speeds Maximized with Simple-Spring Stance Mechanics?". J Appl Physiol, 2014, Vol 117(6), pp 604–615.

Edouard P, et al, "Sprinting: A Potential Vaccine for Hamstring Injury?". Science Performance and Science Reports, 2019.

Ingber D E, "The Architecture of Life". Sci Am, 1998, Vol 278(1), pp 48–57.

Järvinen M J, Lehto M U, "The Effects of Early Mobilisation and Immobilisation on the Healing Process Following Muscle Injuries". Sports Med, 1993, Vol 15(2), pp 78–89.

Kawakami Y, et al, "In vivo Muscle Fiber Behavior During Counter-Movement Exercise in Humans Reveals a Significant Role for Tendon Elasticity". J Physiol, 2002, Vol 540(Pt 2), pp 635–346.

Kram R, Dawson, T J, "Energetics and Biomechanics of Locomotion by Red Kangaroos (Macropus rufus)". Comp Biochem Physiol B Biochem Mol Biol, 1998, Vol 120(1), pp 41–49.

Maas H, Sandercock T G, "Force Transmission between Synergistic Skeletal Muscles through Connective Tissue". J Biomed Biotechnol, 2010, Article ID 575672.

Naito K, Takagi, K, Maruyama, T, "Mechanical Work, Efficiency and Energy Redistribution Mechanisms in Baseball Pitching". J Sports Technol, 2011, Vol 4(1–2), pp 48–64.

Pollack G H, "Cells, Gels, and the Engines of Life. A New, Unifying Approach to Cell Function". Ebner and Sons Publishers, Seattle, Washington, 2001.

Sawicki G S, Lewis, C L, Ferris, D P, "It Pays to Have a Spring in Your Step". Department of Ecology and Evolutionary Biology, Brown University. Exerc Sport Sci Rev, 2009, Vol 37 (3), pp 130–138.

Schleip R, "Fascia as A Sensory Organ: Clinical Applications". Terra Rosa, 2017, Issue 20.

Schleip R, Müller, D G, "Training Principles for Fascial Connective Tissues: Scientific Foundation and Suggested Practical Appli-cations". J Body Mov Ther, 2013, Vol 17(1), pp 103–115.

Weisenthal B M, et al, "Injury Rate and Patterns Among CrossFit Athletes". Orthop J Sports Med, 2014, Vol 2(4), April.

Wiesinger H-P, et al, "Sport-Specific Capacity to Use Elastic Energy in the Patellar and Achilles Tendons of Elite Athletes". Front Physiol, 2017, Vol 8(132).

Zügel M, et al, "Fascial Tissue Research in Sports Medicine: From Molecules to Tissue Adaptation, Injury and Diagnostics. British Journal of Sports Medicine". Br J Sports Med, 2018, Vol 52(23), p 1497.

* A modified version of this chapter was published in Schleip et al., *Fascia in Sport and Movement*, Second Edition, Handspring Publishing, Edinburgh 2020.

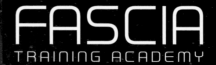

The future is fascial!

Are you convinced? I hope so, because I am sure that everyone, regardless of age and health, will benefit in everyday life from targeted fascia training and more creative movement. If you prefer to practice in a group rather than exercising alone, you can contact the Fascial Fitness Association (FFA), which I co-founded. There are now several thousand FFA-trained fascia trainers around the world who work in their own studios, plus a further training program for those interested in obtaining a training licence. Under 'Find a trainer' on the FFA website, there is a search function that you can use to find certified trainers in your area.

If you want to learn more about fascia training or would prefer to practice under supervision, you can search for a studio near you. The important thing is that you have fun in working toward your goal of feeling fit and making your movements more supple and, as I like to say, more fascia! Regular group training can be very helpful, along with one-on-one coaching from an experienced fascia trainer. This is especially beneficial for beginners and the elderly.

I would like to finish off by taking a look towards the future. I believe that, when it comes to fascial health, there are also implications for health policy. We hinted at this in Chapter 2, when we discussed outdoor exercise areas for adults – 'adult playgrounds', we might say. Adults in particular need to exercise more and move in more varied and thus more fascia-friendly ways, and making this fun and playful is a great way to motivate people. Perhaps the trend toward adult playgrounds will inspire their inclusion in general health programs in the future, and communities will provide playgrounds for all generations. This is by no means a utopian fantasy, but a real opportunity for our industrial nations to show people more ways of having fun and staying in good shape. This will help combat a variety of health problems, including joint disease, back pain, arthritis and obesity – all of which cost governments billions every year.

Nowadays, fascia training and objective views of the fascia in sport and medicine are becoming absolutely essential – and this is just the beginning. The Fascia Research Group, myself included, at the University of Ulm, is planning scientific studies on the effectiveness of a series of fascial exercises, which will include both sport-related aspects and back pain. The group collaborates with sports scientists from other national and international universities, and we are very excited to learn the outcome of the studies. I can say with confidence that this will help us to improve our practices and methods, which will be of great benefit not only to various different sports and types of training, but particularly to the medical sector – and, more specifically, in rehabilitation and prevention.

At this point, I would like to refer again to the somewhat controversial ideas of the great ape researcher Colin Alexander, about whom I may have raved a little in the second chapter (page 93). At the end of his life, Alexander frequently asked one key question: Is it possible that, in our modern civilisation, we not only need official measures to protect animal welfare, but also to protect human welfare, too? Is it not the case that most of us spend our day-to-day lives in our own sort of cage – so far removed from the primitive physical needs of our species – gradually letting our musculoskeletal systems wither away?

Of course, it would be very difficult to impose sanctions on parents who don't give their children adequate freedom to run about. But maybe we should think about introducing some kind of 'Ministry for Movement', so to speak – an organisation that might, for example, randomly check the movement behaviour of employees in a company and, if necessary, release a group of lively fascia therapists to whisk them away to the nearest playground!

I'm not being entirely serious, of course, but it does make me very happy to see that there are currently several interesting new approaches in the field of fascia-friendly healthcare. For example, in recent years, the body therapist and fascia trainer Divo Gitta Müller has developed a special fascia movement program for women, which she offers at her studio in Munich. In addition to addressing muscle stiffening and shortening, a special focus is put on firming up areas of loose tissue. The visible and tangible rejuvenating effects of these exercises are not only apparent in a physical sense, but she and her participants also report feeling overall more youthful, more vibrant and happier in their day-to-day lives.

This is especially good news for me in particular, because I have been married to Divo Gitta Müller for the last 10 years! I would therefore like to start by thanking my wonderful wife for all the inspiring ideas, all the emotional support, and all the many years of fruitful collaboration that we have shared.

I am also grateful to my team in the Fascia Research Group at the University of Ulm, to my long-standing teaching colleagues at the International Rolf Institute in Boulder, Colorado, and here in Europe, as well as the enthusiastic team of trainers at the Fascial Fitness Association.

For this book in particular, however, I must give very special thanks to riva Verlag, who had the idea and, after several attempts, successfully persuaded me to write this book. Finally, I would like to express my unparalleled appreciation to my co-author, the science journalist Johanna Bayer. With her reports for ARD and WDR, she brought the topic of fascia into the spotlight of the German media in 2012, and in doing so succeeded in conveying the fascinating world of fascia to audiences far and wide. Since then, with our books *Fascial Fitness* (2014) and *Fascial Strength Training* (2016), as well as this expanded and revised edition, she has ensured – with all her great expertise and brilliance – that we could walk the fine line between general readability and scientific accuracy. For this, I am truly grateful to her.

About the authors

Robert Schleip

is one of the leading fascia researchers worldwide. He holds a doctorate in human biology and is a certified Rolfing practitioner and psychologist. As a scientist at the University of Ulm, he leads the fascia research group, and also works as a manual Rolfing therapist at his own private practice. In a teaching capacity, he gives lectures on physiotherapy, osteopathy and exercise science. He collaborates with scientists and therapists in a global network of research concerning connective tissue.

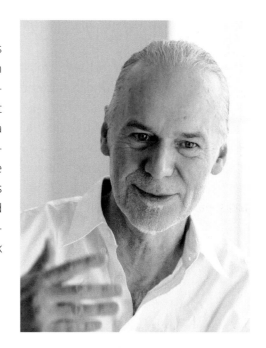

Johanna Bayer

is a science journalist and writer for television broadcasting at major German television channels ARD, WDR and Arte, and also for consumer magazines. She regularly writes about medical topics, including muscles and mobility, neuroscience and anthropology, as well as nutrition, which is the subject of her multi-award-winning blog "Quark und so". Since 2009, she has been involved in researching fascia and its implications for training, everyday life and the treatment of pain, and has reported on these issues in television programs and news articles.

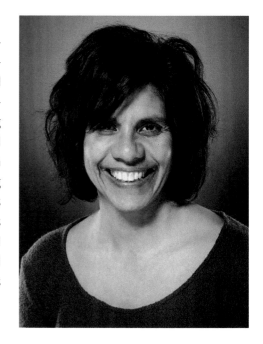

Bill Parisi

is the founder and CEO of the Parisi Speed School franchise and author of *Fascia Training: A Whole-System Approach*. With an international team of coaches and facilities in more than 100 locations worldwide, the Parisi Speed School has trained more than 650,000 athletes between the ages of seven and 18 and produced first-round draft picks in every professional sport – including more than 145 NFL draft picks – and a host of Olympic medallists and champion UFC fighters.

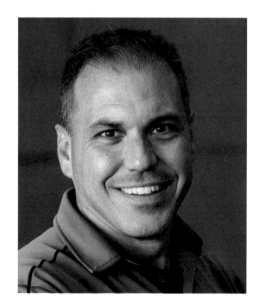

Johnathon Allen

is a writer, photographer and coauthor of *Fascia Training: A Whole-System Approach*. His work has appeared in *Bicycling*, *Outside*, *Adventure Journal*, *Decline* and other publications. He is also author of the nonfiction books *Ray's* and *Doppelganger Effect*.

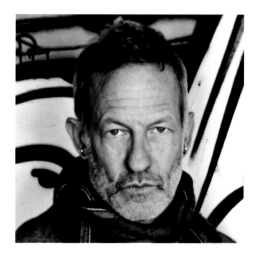

Further reading, additional links and recommended suppliers

Reading recommendations

Dalton, Erik: *Dynamic Body – Exploring Form, Expanding Function*. Freedom From Pain Institute, Oklahoma 2011.

Galloway, Jeff: *The Run-Walk-Run Method* Meyer & Meyer, Aachen 2016

Lesondak, David; Akey, Angeli Maun: *Fascia, Function and Medical Application*. CRC Press, Boca Raton FL 2021

Müller, Divo, Hertzer, Karin: *Train Your Fascia – Tone Your Body*. Meyer & Meyer Sport 2017

Myers, Thomas: *Anatomy Trains – Myofascial Meridians for Manual and Movement Therapists*, 3rd edition, Elsevier, Munich 2015

Parisi, Bill; Allen, Johnathon: *Fascia Training: A Whole-System Approach*. Parisi Media Productions 2019

Pischinger, Alfred; Heine, Hartmut: *The Extracellular Matrix and Ground Regulation: Basis for a Holistic Biological Medicine*. North Atlantic Books, Berkerley CA 2007.

Schleip, Robert; Baker, Amanda: *Fascia in Sport and Movement*, Handspring Publishing Limited, 2015

Schleip, Robert, et al. (eds.): *Fascia: The Tensional Network of the Human Body: The science and clinical applications in manual and movement therapy*. Elsevier, Edinburgh 2012

Wilke, Jan; Krause, Frieder; Vogt, Lutz; Banzer, Winfried: *What is evidence-based about myofascial chains: a* systematic review, *Arch. of Physical Medicine and Rehabilitation, 97(3);* pp.454–461, Saunders, WB.

Additional links and resources

Online Fascial Fitness certification courses, fascia-focused sports and movement training modules, fascia dissection courses, expert interviews, recent research findings, instructor directories.
Fascia Training Academy:
fasciatrainingacademy.com

An international, evidence-based curriculum for speed training and athletic performance.
Parisi Speed School:
parisischool.com

Loaded movement training tools, educational resources, exercise videos.
ViPR PRO:
vipr.com

Photo credits

Adobe Stock/zstock: 25
Barto: 116, left
Beate Michalke/www.beate-michalke.de: 9
BLACKROLL©Sebastian Schöffel: 247, 250 2nd from top, 250 3rd from top, 250 2nd from bottom, 251 1st from bottom, 251 2nd from bottom
Collage using images from Shutterstock: 258
Dr Christian Schmelzer, Dr Andrea Heinz, Institut für Angewandte Dermatopharmazie (Institute for Applied Dermapharmacology) at the Martin Luther University of Halle-Wittenberg, Halle (Saale): 27 right, 81
Courtesy of Endovivo Productions and Dr J. Guimberteau: 17
European Rolfing Association e. V.: 45, 239
fascialnet.com: 12, 33, 37 top, 80
fle.xx Rückgratkonzept GmbH, fle-xx.com: 251 2nd from top
Fotografie Meyer im Hagen/Hamburg: 8
Fotolia: adimas: 38; bilderzwerg: 144
Getty Images: Mark Wieland: 84; Steve Schapiro: 58
Hermann Baumann, Berlin, by: Medau, Hinrich: *Deutsche Gymnastik. Lehrweise Medau*, Union Deutsche Verlagsgesellschaft, Stuttgart, 1940: 77
imago/Ulmer: 16
iStockphoto/Lorado: 98
Courtesy of Karger Publishers, image modified based on Nishimura et al. 1994 (Acta Anat. 151: 250–257): 37 bottom
Kristin Hoffmann, based on an illustration from: Rode, Christian (2010): Interaction Between Passive and Contractile Muscle Elements: Re-evaluation and New Mechanisms, PhD thesis, Jena, Germany, see also: http://wiki.ifs-tud.de/_media/biomechanik/projekte/interaktion_zwischen_passiven_und_kontraktilen_muskelelementen_neubewertung_und_neue_mechanismen_von_dr._christian_rode.pdf, based on an illustration from: Hill, A. V.: *The heat of shortening and the dynamic constants of muscle*. Proceedings of the Royal Society of London: Series B, 1938, 126, 136–195: 62
Kristin Hoffmann: 30, 63, 69 right, 70, 146
Leni Riefenstahl © Archiv Leni LRP: 76 bottom left, bottom right
PINO Pharmazeutische Präparate GmbH, www.pinoshop.de: 250, 4th from top
riva Verlag, in line with shutterstock/Soul wind: 114, 118 bottom
riva Verlag: 29, 115, 117, 118 top, 120 et seq., 123 et seq., 126 et seq., 191, 241, 251 3rd from top
courtesy of Robert Schleip, modified based on: Kawakami, Y, Muraoka, T, Ito, S, Kaneshisa, H, Fukunaga, T (2002): *In Vivo Muscle Fibre Behaviour during Countermovement Exercise in Humans Reveals a Significant Role for Tendon Elasticity*. J Physiol 540 (2): 635–646: 87 et seq.
courtesy of Robert Schleip, modified based on: Reeves, ND, Narici, MV, Maganaris, CN (2006): *Myotendinous Plasticity to Ageing and Resistance Exercise in Humans*. In: Exp Physiol 91(3): 483–498: 79 top
Robert Schleip: 21
Schelke Fotografie: 10, 269 top
Schünke M, Schulte E, Schumacher U et al., ed. Prometheus LernAtlas der Anatomie. *Allgemeine Anatomie und Bewegungssystem*. 4th edition, Thieme, Stuttgart 2014, Fig. 1.9 B, p. 118, illustration by Karl Wesker: 55
ScienceFoto.de/Dr. André Kempe: 27, left
Shutterstock.com: Andrey Plis: 104; Andrey_Popov: 53; AntonMaltsev: 86; Barber 6: 64 left; bitt24: 256; chaoss: 19; Claire Lucia: 60; De Visu: 95; Digital Genetics: 72 et seq., 75; dlodewijks: 64 right; eastern light photography: 83 right; Elena Schweitzer: 264; fizkes: 141, 234; george green: 65; iLight photo: 246; Jose Gil: 116 right; KieferPix: 259; Kingapl: 261; Lapina: 59; leonori/edited by Manuela Amode: 257; Maridav: 83 left; mokokomo: 68; Nanette Grebe: 237; Petar Djordjevic: 236; ProSha: 69 left; Radu Razvan/edited by Maria Wittek: 220; Rawpicel.com: 100; Samo Trebizan: 92; Scott Tomer: 93; SJ Allen: 66; snapgalleria: 52; stihii: 61; Suzanne Tucker: 96; Syda Productions: 232; topseller: 31; Valeria Aksakova: 263; VIZAPHOTO PHOTOGRAPHER: 255
Springer Science + Business Media based in Järvinen, Tero A. H.: *Organization and Distribution of Intramuscular Connective Tissue in Normal and Immobilized Skeletal Muscles*. In: Journal of Muscle Research and Cell Motility, Jan. 2002, fig. 6: 79 bottom
Tittel, Kurt: *Beschreibende und funktionelle Anatomie*, 15th edition, Kiener Verlag, Munich 2012, p. 273: 76, top left
Tittel, Kurt: *Beschreibende und funktionelle Anatomie*, 15th edition, Kiener Verlag, Munich 2012, p. 324: 76 top right
TOGU GmbH, www.togu.de: 250 3rd from bottom, 4th from bottom
TRJavelin [CC BY-SA 4.0 (https://creativecommons.org/licenses/by-sa/4.0)], from Wikimedia Commons: 82
Vukašin Latinović: 103, 107, 109, 111 et seq., 133 et seq., 137, 143, 145, 147, 149, 151, 153, 155, 157, 159, 161, 163, 165 et seq., 169, 170 et seq., 173, 175 et seq., 179, 181 et seq., 184 et seq., 187 et seq., 190, 192 et seq., 196 et seq., 200 et seq., 203 et seq., 206 et seq., 209, 212 et seq., 215 et seq., 218 et seq., 221 et seq., 224 et seq., 227, 250 1st from top, 1st from bottom, 251 1st from top, 269 bottom
www.bv-osteopathie.de, Bundesverband Osteopathie e. V., BVO. 240
courtesy of www.eden-reha.de: 7

Overview of exercises

The basic program **142–155**
  Rolling out the feet .... from 144
  Elastic jumps for the calves and Achilles tendon .... from 146
  Stretching the front and rear lines: eagle flight .... from 148
  Stretching the waist and sides: eagle wings on a chair .... from 150
  Activating the shoulders and shoulder girdle: spring-backs using
  the arms .... from 152
  Relaxing the neck and back: snake dance .... from 154

Exercises for problem areas: back, neck, arms, hips
and feet **156–190**
  A short program for back problems **157–167**
  Rolling out the lumbar fascia .... from 158
  Stretching the back: cat .... from 160
  African bends .... from 162
  Flying sword .... from 164
  Relieving the spinal chain .... from 166

  Office pains: problems in the neck, arms and shoulders **168–175**
  Stretching the shoulders 170
  Freeing up the neck 171
  Relaxation for tired forearms .... from 172
  Momentum for the whole body: swinging bamboo .... from 174

  The hip area **176–182**
  Rolling out the outer thighs 177
  Activating the outer thighs .... from 178
  Swinging the legs .... from 180
  The skate 182

  For the feet and gait **183–190**
  Rolling out the plantar fascia 185
  Sensitising the soles of the feet .... from 186
  Swinging the legs 188
  Elastic jumps for the feet, calves and Achilles tendon 189
  Stretching the Achilles tendon 190

For Vikings, contortionists and crossover types **191–198**

    Vikings with firm connective tissue **192–194**

        Opening up the rib cage 193

        Flying sword 194

    Contortionists with soft connective tissue . . . . **from 195**

        For the chest and shoulders: firming the bust 196

    Crossover types 197

        Stretching the Achilles tendon 197

        Rolling out the lumbar fascia 198

Different exercises for men and women **199–209**

    Exercises and tips for women **200–203**

        Rolling out the thighs 201

        Tightening the thighs and buttocks 202

        Tightening the tummy 203

    Exercises and tips for men **204–209**

        The flamingo . . . . from 205

        Throwing 207

        Stretching the adductors . . . . from 208

Exercises for athletes **210–220**

    Sport-specific fascial care 211

    Self-help for sore muscles **212–216**

        Rolling out the calves 213

        Rolling out other parts of the body to relieve muscle soreness . . . . from 214

        Slow stretching for muscle soreness: elephant step 216

    Balancing exercises for runners **217–219**

        Stretching the Achilles tendon 218

        Running variations 219

    Tips for cyclists 220

**Everyday life as an exercise: making your movements
more creative** **221–224**

        Stair dance 222

        Light switch Kung Fu 223

        African bends in everyday life 224

Guidelines for the elderly **221–227**

        Swinging bamboo 226

        Flying sword 227

Index

A

Abdomen 35
    lower 165, 196, 216
Abdominal
    cavity 25, 35, 38, 46
    core 75
    fascia 24
    muscles 54, 75, 203, 241
    network 75
    tension 75
Achilles tendon 64, 65, 66, 72, 87, 96, 107,
    144, 146, 183, 189, 217, 255
    rupture 146
Activation 142
Acupuncture 48, 231, 237, 245
    points 238
    sham 238
Adductor 81, 208
Adductors–pelvic floor line 74
Adipocyte 32
Aerobic 58
African bends 97, 162, 224
Age 19, 24, 32, 63, 78, 91, 93, 124, 132,
    136, 225
Ageing 59, 78, 93
Age-related stiffness 59
Alexander, Colin F. 93
Amateur athletes 58
Amino acids 256, 259
Anatomy 38, 43, 47, 70, 95, 242
    fascial 7
Ankle 75
Anxiety disorder 50, 94
Aorta 31
Aponeurosis 61
Arm(s) 74, 156, 168, 169
    –abdomen line 174
    –chest–abdomen line 73, 150, 164
Arthritis 91, 92, 94, 255, 266

B

Back 132, 156
    bone 71
    complaints 55, 97
    exercises, conventional 104
    fascia 53, 54, 75, 162
    fascia, deep 40, 48, 233
    fascia, large 24, 38, 54
    hollow 117
    massage 251
    pain 17, 20, 40, 50, 53, 97, 104, 137, 148,
        157, 164, 234, 235, 255, 266
    pain research 54
    problem 94
    program 157
    relaxation 154
    stretches 114, 160
Balance 92, 183
Ball 96, 133, 144, 203, 207, 251
    double 166, 251
    rubber 65, 147
    tennis 133, 144, 214
Balloon 171, 203
Barefoot 20, 119, 136, 146, 180, 189, 222
Basic
    communication 110
    fascia 33, 102, 139
    function 33, 102, 106, 110
    movements 99
    moving 106
    program 142
    regulation 44
    shaping 103
    supply 108
    training 102
Blackroll 135
    training 172
Bladder 31
Blockade 45, 231
Blood
    circulation 233, 236, 245

pressure 40, 41, 44, 46, 104, 233, 235, 239, 242
sugar 262
-thinning medications 137
vessel 29, 30, 39, 43, 108, 248, 254, 263
Blueroll 135
Body
awareness 21, 42, 50, 110, 136, 183, 217
fluid 32
parts, sensitive 250
perception 41, 101, 110, 137, 195
posture 49, 71, 91
therapy 16, 20, 45, 238, 267
type 25, 30
Bones 27, 34, 36, 38, 59, 61, 62, 68, 70, 91, 99, 242, 254
attachment point 38
tissue 62
Bove, Geoffrey 48, 237
Bowen therapy 244
Brain 40, 235
lining 31
Breathing
mindful 140
patterns 138
relaxed 141
Building blocks
fascial 26
Buttocks, tightening 202

C

Calcium 27
Calf 72, 114, 143, 146, 189, 197, 213, 220
aponeurosis 146
muscle 87
Callanetics 58
Capsules 70
injury 81
Cardiac
arrest 91, 263
function 235

Cartilage 25, 32, 55, 62, 70, 92, 176
damage 255
Catapult
effect 64, 180
mechanism 66
Cell 28, 32, 44, 47, 48, 53, 117, 254
connective tissue 28, 30, 62, 78, 259
contractile 53
fat 28, 32
growth 258
immune 28, 34
inflammatory 234
lymph 28, 30
metabolism 29, 34, 257, 258
muscle 39, 47, 62
nerve 60
wall 39
Cellulite 115, 117, 200, 221, 247, 254
Cervical
chain 178
muscles 166
spine 171
Chapelle, Susan 48, 237
Chest 114
muscles 118, 152, 196
tightening 196
Children 138
Chin to chest test 126
Chiropractic 49
Circulatory problems 248
Climbing 94
Clothing 19, 136
Collagen 26, 28, 32, 39, 55, 63, 78, 258, 260
bundle 31
content 31
fibres 27, 28, 29, 32, 45, 61, 63, 86
production 86, 195, 257
synthesis 117, 257, 258, 264
Communicating 33, 34, 102, 110, 139
Communication phenomenon 34

Complaints 53, 90, 103, 104, 246, 263
   arms and shoulders 97
   characteristic 115
Connective tissue 11, 16, 19, 24, 31, 32, 34, 36,
   38, 40, 48, 50, 70, 100, 148, 199, 247, 259,
   262, 265
   care 255
   cells 28, 29, 30, 62, 78, 86, 195, 256, 259
   collagen production 257
   condition 20, 90
   disorders 20, 117, 119
   fibres 28, 80
   fibrous 26, 30
   firm 113, 118, 190, 258
   functions 26
   intramuscular 105
   knots 117
   loose 29, 30
   massage 46
   matted 59
   matting 192
   muscular 220
   nutrition 254
   points 238
   soft 113, 115, 117, 196, 236
   structure 114
   training 78
   types 19, 28, 33, 60, 106, 113, 118,
     191, 199
   weak 116, 139
Continuum distortion 242
Contortionist 113, 114, 116, 139, 235, 236
   exercises 195
   features 117, 121
   test 120
Contraction 39, 62, 65
Coordination 18, 19, 42, 71, 78, 86, 90, 92, 94,
   113, 192, 193, 225, 241
Core 241
Crossover type 114, 198
   exercises 197
   features 118
   test 126
   weaknesses 126

Cuff weight 133, 196, 202
Cyclist 213, 220
Cylinder distortion 242

D

Dancer 77, 86, 91
Dancing 91, 117, 189
Degeneration 55, 91, 97, 99
Dementia 91
Depression 49, 50, 91, 113, 263
Depth perception 41, 112
Dermatome 238
Dexterity 92
Diabetes 91, 262
Diagnosis, medical 119
Diagonal torso line 73, 174, 183
Dicke, Elisabeth 43, 46
Digestion 235
Disc injury 17
   exercising 146
   jogging 95
   running 95, 146, 189
   slipped 55, 115, 137, 164, 255
Disorder 53, 59, 90, 144
   anatomical 242
   circulatory 248
   connective tissue 20, 117
   fascia 35
   lymphatic 109
   muscular 53
   psychological 113
   regulatory 239
Dopamine 101
Dorsal line 144, 148, 164, 220
   functional 72
   large 54, 72
Double ball 166, 251
Drinking 255
Dumbbell 88, 133, 174, 192
Dynamic functions 71

E

Eagle flight 148
Eagle wings 150

Earlobes, attached 118
Ehlers-Danlos syndrome 116
Elasticity 28, 85, 204
    elastic 63, 105
Elastin 26, 27, 28, 31, 39
    fibres 27, 29, 32, 258
    springs 146
Elbow 120
    problems 20, 90
Elderly people 225
Embodiment 110
Endomysium 37, 62, 88
Energy
    flow 45, 238
    kinetic 64
    transfer 36, 61, 78
Enzymatic crosslinks 258
Enzymes 28
Epimysium 37, 62, 84, 85, 89
Everyday
    immobility 92
    movement 58, 97, 107, 119
Exercises 132
    springing 106
Exercise mat 136
    Extension 146

F
Fascia(l) 7, 10, 16, 24, 31, 38, 61, 78, 86, 100,
    146, 158, 231
    ageing 79
    architecture of 80
    band 61, 242
    blaster 243, 247
    components 25, 26
    condition 19, 90
    crossing points 48, 237
    distortion model 242, 243
    elastic storage capacity 210
    exercises 78, 132
    experts 49, 55
    fibres 88
    fitness 59, 254
    Fitness Association 17, 132, 266

functions 100, 102
health 258
importance 18, 41, 52
injury 17, 265
lata 80, 95
layer 32, 36, 39, 54
leg, 108
line 18, 60, 67, 71, 74–77, 85, 101, 107, 132,
    142, 148, 168, 174, 183, 239, 242
lumbar 48, 50, 53, 67, 97, 114, 118, 157,
    160, 162, 164, 255
    thickened 78
    rolling out 158
mechanics 67
mechanism 64
musculoskeletal system 25, 36
matting 78
network 18, 26, 54, 71, 81, 100,
    132, 138
neurotransmitters 47
objectives 85
older people, and 225
organs, of the 41
physiological functions 34
Releazer 243, 247
renewal 108
researcher 11, 17, 32, 43
Research Project 47
Research Team 10
roller 135, 136, 243, 247
rolling out 136, 247
sensor 41
sheath 36, 37, 41, 55, 62 63, 84, 85, 146,
    240, 242, 245
sheets 25, 38
specialists 230
stretching 192
structure 91
system 20, 59
therapy using tools 246
thigh, 80, 108
tissue 24, 27, 36, 60, 61, 78, 90, 102
training 11, 17, 18, 58, 80, 81, 85, 90, 101,
    113, 199, 211, 258, 266

treatment 41, 49, 110, 243
units 70
Fallen angel test 128
Fat 114, 254
cell 28, 32
deposit 200
Fatty tissue 25, 32, 254
Feeling 40, 101, 102, 110, 112, 113, 138, 139, 183, 192, 195, 197, 225
Feldenkrais teacher 230
Femur 71
Fibres 25, 26, 28, 31, 37, 39, 55, 61, 78, 86, 88, 256, 265
bundles 36, 37, 61, 78
Fibroblast 28
Fibromatosis 117
Fibrous protein 28
Fill tissue 25, 35
Findley, Thomas 49
Fitness, mental 92
Flexibility 27, 204
Fluid
absorption 255
congestion 220
content 28, 29, 32
exchange 86, 100, 108, 109, 112, 158, 231, 236, 240, 248
system 240
Foam roller 100, 108, 135
Folding distortion 242
agglutinations 48, 237
healthy 81, 90
interoceptors 50
mechanical properties 112
muscle soreness 85
shortened 148
supply to 109
Foot 75, 144, 156, 183, 189
exercises 142
problems 20
rolling 148
sole of the 72, 75, 142, 144, 145, 184
Forearms 172
Forward fold test 120, 123
Front line 73

Frozen shoulder 90, 117, 152
Function
sensory 100
Functional dorsal line 72
Functional front line 73
Fuse 61
Fusing 35

G
Gait 53, 67, 71, 91, 156, 162, 183, 189, 234
Gall bladder 31
Ganten, Detlev 91
Gibson, William 84
Girdle, fascial 75
Golgi receptors 39, 245
Graven-Nielsen, Thomas 84
Gravity 65, 91, 107
Green tea powder 265
Grip, osteopathic 110
Ground substance 26, 28, 30, 32, 100
Growth
hormone 259
impulse 88
Gymnastics 39, 77, 230, 233
exercises for preventing back problems 54

H
Hands behind your back 122
Hand syndrome 117
Hard foam roller 135
Harmony, disturbed 231
Head 38, 67, 154, 171
Headache 20, 154
Head, Henry 46
Healing 18, 94, 105, 230
Health insurance company 104, 240
Heart rate, increased 41
Heel 32, 144, 147
cushion 72, 185, 246
spur 20, 90, 96, 144
Hips 29, 75, 86, 94, 132, 150, 156, 176, 188, 204, 220
joint 19, 90, 144, 148
operation 176

Homeopathy 49
Hopping 65, 87, 106, 189
Hormone 113, 236, 254
    function 258
    growth 259
    thyroid 258
Huijing, Peter 48
Hyaluronan 29
Hyaluronic acid 29
Hydration 255
Hypermobile 117, 122
Hypermobility, pathological 116

I

Illness 136
Imbalance 119
Immobility 59, 78, 91
Immune
    cell 28, 30, 34
    defence 44
    system 28, 42, 257, 263, 265
Increased performance 18
Inflammation 53, 82, 84, 91, 96, 104, 105, 136,
    144, 233, 254, 263
Inflammatory
    cells 234
    neurotransmitter 108, 245
    substances 236
Insula 50, 52
Insulin
    production 257
    resistance 262
International Fascia Research Congress 26
Interoception 50
Interstitial receptors 39
Intervertebral discs 19, 29, 50, 53, 55, 90,
    146, 259
    degenerative 91

J

Janda type 119
Jogging 66, 89, 146, 247
Joint(s) 40, 42, 60, 70, 101, 116, 195, 221
    arthritis 261
    capsules 25, 211

disease (degenerative) 93, 266
dislocation 121
flexible 114
function 50
inflammation 92
injury 81
instability 236
layer of cartilage 94
overweight 254
painful 91
proprioceptive awareness 121
range of motion 92
signs of degeneration 99
stability 113, 117
strain 94
stress 80
Jump(s) 65
    elastic 189
    fascial 146
Jumping 65, 87, 189
    force 105
    performance 260

K

Keyhole surgery 35
Kidney 31, 32
Kinetic
    energy 27, 63, 107
    momentum 207
Klingler, Werner 35
Knee 29, 32, 94, 120, 176, 200
    bend 108
    joint 74, 220
    pain 237
    to forehead test 124
    to wall test 127

L

Laban, Rudolf von 241
Langevin, Helene 48, 233, 237
Large dorsal line 72
Lateral line 75, 150
Leg 54, 67, 72, 75, 136, 148, 160, 168, 180,
    188, 190, 204, 217, 248, 254
    stretching 205

Lehmann-Horn, Frank 47
Lieberman, Daniel 95
Ligamentous apparatus 176
Ligaments 19, 25, 31, 38, 42, 55, 69, 70, 77, 81,
    90, 94, 99, 176, 211, 242, 254
Light switch Kung Fu 223
Lipid metabolism disorder 262
Long holds 59, 152, 168
Loss of motion 126, 136, 176
Lower back pain 71, 90, 168
Lumbar spine 117, 239
Lungs 31, 235
Lymph 34, 108, 248
Lymphatic congestion 136, 248
Lymphatic disorder 109
Lymph cell 28, 30
Lymph nodes 32
Lymph system 109

M

Magnesium 258
    symptoms of deficiency 91, 257
Man 114, 117, 119, 132, 193, 199, 204,
    208, 258
Manual therapist 7
Marfan syndrome 116
Massage 41, 46, 48, 49, 51, 108, 212, 230, 236
    holds 238
Massaging 101
Matrix 28, 29, 44, 78
Mechanoreceptor 39, 50, 110
    golgi receptors 39
    interstitial receptors 39
    Pacinian corpuscles 39
    Ruffini corpuscles 39
Mechanosensor 144
Medau, Hinrich and Senta 77
Meditation 104, 231, 233, 234
Meinl, Daniela 132
Mense, Siegfried 47
Meridian 45, 48, 231, 237
Metabolism 30, 33, 34, 80, 88, 89, 94,
    109, 144, 192, 225, 231, 236, 240,
    254, 257

Metabolic
    activation 251
    disorder 91
    factor 82
    function 34
    residue 236
    stimulation 250
    waste 108
Metabolite 44, 108
Method, alternative 231
Michalsen, Andreas 233
Micro-injury 53
Minerals 265
Minimally invasive 35
Misuse 91
Mixed type 114, 126
Mobility 12, 17, 39, 59, 86, 110, 113, 144, 154,
    166, 192, 208, 211, 225, 238, 240, 254
    hips 176
    joints 60
    lack of 32, 54, 91, 110
    legs 202
    limited 148
    mechanical 235
Mobility, low 113, 118
Mobility, high 113, 117
Motion
    blindness 43
    perception 41, 211
    sensor 30, 41, 42, 112, 266
Motor neuron 40
Move 33, 43, 102, 106, 139
Movement 8, 18, 21, 30, 33, 39, 40, 41, 42, 51,
    58, 60, 62, 67, 71, 76, 90, 95, 100, 108, 110,
    113, 121, 221, 230, 239, 245, 266
    feeling 41
    forms of 92
    functional 18
    human 91
    impulses 205
    in everyday life 58
    patterns 92, 94, 97, 101, 207
    processes 19, 90
    repertoire 91, 97

sensation 21
springing 107
too little 262
training exercises 98, 144
variations 189
Movement control, internal 42
Müller, Divo Gitta 267
Multi-directional 31
Multiple sclerosis 94
Musculoskeletal stress 99
Musculoskeletal system 25, 26, 35, 36, 38, 40,
    48, 60, 221, 235
Muscle
    aches 260
    bundle 25
    cell 39, 47, 62, 80
    chain 18, 205
    contraction 89
    direction 86
    disorder 53
    fascia 24, 33, 37, 40, 63, 81, 86, 106
    fibre 26, 36, 37, 39, 50, 82, 87, 88, 89,
        211, 245
    fibril 83
    insertions 242
    movement 40
    problem 17, 210
    self-help 212
    sheath 50, 211
    soreness 17, 82, 84, 100, 110, 210, 213,
        214, 216
    strength 115
    tendons 50
    tension 40, 43, 68, 88, 89, 101
    tissue 17, 37, 84, 88, 220
    tone 68, 110, 245
    training 21, 85, 138, 200
Muscles 19, 51, 78, 90, 114
    incorrectly exercised 53
    pelvic- 203, 241
    shoulder and neck 94
Musculofascial chain 66
Musculofascial unit 67, 85
Myers, Thomas 31, 49, 67, 71, 73

Myofascial
    hardenings 246
    line 71
    meridians 49
    release 110
    structure 97
Myofibroblast 48, 117

N
Natural remedies 230
Neck 114, 118, 132, 154, 156, 168,
    169, 200
    fascia 95, 154
    pain 20, 90, 117, 154
    relaxing 154
Nerve cells 60
Nerve endings 29, 30, 39, 40, 41, 42, 238
Nervous system 40, 41, 45, 47, 231, 233
    autonomous 41, 141
    central 39
    vegetative 40, 41, 46, 51, 110, 235
Network 26, 30, 34, 67, 71
    abdominal 75
    dynamic 71
    fascial 18, 49, 54, 70, 156, 240
    signal 48
    structure 78, 85
Neurotransmitter 28, 32, 47, 48, 101, 113,
    235, 236, 254
Neural
    circuit 245
    control 18
    fibres 40
    pathway 42
    reflexes 240
Neurological disorders 137
Neurologist 40
Neurology 47
Neuron 40, 42
Nicotine 254
Nordic walking poles 146
Nutrient exchange 34
Nutrition 21, 254, 260, 262, 263
Nutritional supplements 259

O

Organism 24, 44, 51, 91, 199, 259
Organs 110
Orthopaedic 7, 26, 69
Osteopath 20
Osteopathy 43, 49, 51, 231, 239
Osteoporosis 137
Over-the-head movement 94
Overweight 91, 254, 262, 266
Oxygen content 254

P

Pacinian corpuscles 39
Pain 18, 19, 36, 40–42, 55, 90, 91, 110, 117,
    159, 238, 263
    back 17, 50, 53, 97, 148, 157, 234
    development 85
    head 20
    hip 176
    joint 91
    knee 237
    muscle soreness 84
    neck 20, 90, 154
    pressure 84
    problem 59
    receptor 40, 48
    research 84
    sacrum 71, 90, 168
    sensor 53
    shoulder 81
    syndrome 242
    threshold 248
    treatment 233
    when moving 48, 59, 84
Palm 115, 120
Pelvis 46, 73, 114, 166, 182,
    205, 239
Pelvic floor 54, 74, 140, 165
    muscles 203, 241
Pelvic stability 74
Pendulum walk 188
People's illness 53
Perception 50, 121, 138, 211
    exercise 113

internal 34, 41, 50, 195
    refining 251
Perceptual
    stimulation 251
    system 52
Performance 19, 58, 90
    athlete 58
Perimysium 37, 88
Periosteum 38, 61, 257
Phenomenon, interoceptive 235
Phenomenon, proprioceptive 235
Physical movement 17, 110, 242
Physiologist 25, 34, 40
Physiology 40, 47, 237
Pilates 54, 58, 231, 241
    roller 135
Pischinger, Alfred 43, 44
Plantar fascia 66, 72, 75, 95, 96, 144, 185
Plastic bottle 133
Playground 99, 266
Posture 19, 45, 49, 61, 67, 71, 72, 78, 97,
    111,150, 162, 198
    disorder 36
    posture 49
    problems 238
    unilateral 245
Potassium 258
Powerhouse 241
Pregnancy 114
    stretch marks 115
Pre-loading 65, 106
Pressure 30, 39, 41, 49, 50, 51, 100, 108, 110,
    136, 214, 237, 238, 248
    applying 236
    changes 39
    pain under 84
Prevention 58, 267
Problem 20, 53, 59, 90, 103, 117, 132
    areas 19, 132, 156, 199, 247
    athletic 210
    back 94
    back fascia 53
    cartilage 92
    elbow 90

foot 20
  metabolic 91
  muscle 17, 210
  neck 168
  posture 238
  shoulder 20, 90, 117, 152, 168
  wrist 202
Procedure
  complementary 231, 237
  manual 239
  imaging 11
Proprioception 40, 42, 50, 121, 211
Protein 25, 27, 248, 256, 260
Psychological disorder 113
Pulse 104
  slowing of 46

Q

Qigong 231

R

Radicals, free 254, 265
Range of motion 94, 103, 195, 221
  limited 36
Receptor 33, 39, 41, 138, 237
  type 40
Recovery
  alternative 48, 49
  complementary 237
  methods 230
  success 231
Regeneration 18, 81, 85, 86, 105, 141, 211, 225, 243, 248, 251
  time 19, 90
Regulation 43, 51, 262
Regulatory disorder 239, 242
Rehabilitation 58, 241, 267
Rehabilitative gymnastics 77
Resilience 69, 90, 138
Rheumatism 136, 263
Rib cage 193
Röhler, Thomas 82
Rolf, Ida P. 43, 45, 49, 91, 238
Rolfing 45, 49, 110, 237, 238

course of 49
  session 238
  technique 48
  therapist 45, 47, 230, 238, 269
Roller 133, 135, 139, 248
  fascia 135, 136
  foam 100, 108, 135
  hardness 135
Rolling out 214
  the feet 144
Rossmann, Markus 132
Rotational movements 55
Roughage 259, 265
Rubber ball 65
  feeling 153
Ruffini corpuscles 39, 41
Running 59, 65, 146, 219
Runner
  balance exercise 217

S

Sailboat 69
Scar(s) 32, 35, 48, 113, 115, 118, 246
  formation 43
  surgical 36
Sciatic nerve 36, 40
Scoliosis 121
Scurvy 257
Self
  -awareness 113
  -healing 51, 233
  -massage 100, 108, 110, 212
  -perception 40
  -test 60, 119
  -treatment 110
Sensor 17, 30, 33, 39, 41, 85
  fascial 41
  motion 41
  pain 53
  proprioceptive 40
Sensory
  information 101
  organs 39, 100
  perception 101

Sex(es) 124
    the difference between 114, 199
Shaping 33, 34, 102, 103, 139
Sheath 25, 36, 38, 61, 62, 85, 86, 88
Sherman, Karen 234
Shiatsu 231
Shoes 59, 92, 136
Shoulders 29, 74, 96, 118, 143, 152, 168,
    196, 204
    activating 152
    blade stabilisers 114
    complaints 238
    effect 250
    –elbow fascial line 74
    exercise 168
    frozen 20, 117
    girdle, activating 152
    /neck muscles 94
    /neck/arm syndrome 168
    pain 81, 90
    problem 20, 90, 117, 152
    stiffness 97
    stretches 169
Signal network 48
Silicon 259, 260
Sit muscles 118
Sit-up test 127
Skeleton 31, 38, 60, 68
Skin 27, 29, 32, 34, 35, 38, 40, 41, 51, 237
Sleep 254, 259, 264
    disorder 141
    lack of 262
    pattern 235
Smoking 254
Snake dance 71
Spinal chain 71, 158, 166, 171
    relieving the 166
Spinal column 69, 70, 146, 164, 250, 251
Spine 53, 182
    damage 17, 53
    surgery 53, 94
Spiral line 73, 183
Sporting injury 17, 81, 210
Sports science 18
Sports scientist 17, 26, 106, 267

Spring-back motion 106, 152
Springing 62, 64, 77, 102, 106, 112, 137, 139,
    142, 162, 192, 195, 197, 225, 242
Squeezing 250
Stability, high 113
Stair dance 222
Standing 42
Staubesand, Jochen 47
Stecco, Carla 32
Sternum 73
Stiffening 118
Stiffness 18, 125
Still, Andrew Taylor 43, 51, 239
Stimulate 102, 108, 112, 138, 139, 144, 183,
    192, 195, 197, 211
Stimulation 18, 49, 136, 231, 240, 250
Stomach 30, 54, 71, 73, 114, 118, 152, 164,
    171, 194, 227, 254
Storage capacity 28, 66, 67, 85, 183, 210, 211
    elastic 80, 112
    fascial 63, 106
    tendons 66
Straddle 123
Strain 81, 142
    injuries 7, 81, 96, 243
Strength-building 21
Stress 7, 48, 53, 104, 233, 236, 242,
    254, 259
    load 141
    response 34
    stimuli 91
Stretching 39, 41, 58, 88–90, 101–106, 112,
    139, 190, 192, 195, 197, 216, 225, 231,
    235, 241
    back 160
    lateral 150
    passive 89
    position 105, 235
    rocking 106
    shoulders 169
    side 150
    slow 39, 105, 192, 212, 233
    springing 105
    static 105
    strain 31

the lines 148
    yoga 233
Stretch test 121, 128
Stroke 94
Stroking 101
Structural
    actin 39, 83
    collagen 39
    elastin 39
    integration 49
    protein 26, 39, 83
    titin 39, 83
Subcutaneous 31, 114
    connective tissue 50
    tissue 25, 114
Sugar 262
    molecule 28, 29
    types of 262
Superficial frontal arm line 73
Suppleness 204
Supporting tissue 34, 38
Surgery
    abdominal 35
    hip 176
    minimally invasive 35
    spinal 53
Suspension
    dynamic 107
    elastic 87
Swinging 77, 106
    exercises 78
    gymnastics 77
Sympathetic nervous system 104
Synovial fluid 29

I

Tectonic fixation 242
Teirich-Leube, Hede 46
Tendon(s) 19, 25, 31, 33, 36, 38, 40, 42, 63–65,
    70, 81, 86, 87, 90, 106, 146, 211, 245, 254
    catapult effect 65
    insertion 40
    sheath 36
    tissue 62
Tennis ball 133

Tensegrity model 70
Tensile
    direction 31
    elements 71
    energy 65, 106
    force 19, 48, 82, 85, 200, 204
    network 54
    strain 39, 63, 101
    stress 89
    system 69, 166
Tension 16, 20, 33, 34, 41, 49, 62, 64, 70, 89,
    100, 110, 117, 132, 152, 200, 233, 238, 249
    elastic 200
    network 60, 67, 68, 132
Testosterone 258
Therapy, manual 49, 230, 236
Thighs 32, 72, 95, 114, 148, 150, 158, 200,
    202, 214, 220
    outer 177
Thorocolumbar line, diagonal 73
Throwing 97, 207
Thymus gland 32
Thyroid hormone 258
Tissue 35, 63
    fluid 100, 136
    types 30
Torso 54, 71, 72, 73, 97, 122, 164, 168, 178
    muscles 241
    stretch test 123
    twists 55
Tozzi, Paolo 241
Trace element 254, 257, 258, 259
Training
    concept 18
    methods 242
    principles 85, 138
    program 17, 18, 20, 21, 58, 86, 100,
        138, 221
    stimulus 80, 87, 100, 101, 103
    targeted 18, 60
Trigger
    band 242
    point hernia 242
    point treatment 110, 245
Tummy tightener 203

Turmeric 265
Twisting motions 55

U
Underuse 91, 93, 94
Unused arc theory 92

V
Vegetarians 256, 261
Vertebrae 55
Vertebral segments 69
Vikings 113, 115, 139, 190, 236
    disease 115
    exercises 192, 193
    features 118
    men 115
    problems 117
    test 122
    women 114
Vitamin(s) 254, 257, 259, 265

W
Waist stretches 150
Walking 42, 43, 59, 65, 66, 67, 73, 146,
    183, 188
    meditation 188
Warm-up 142
    exercises 138
    massage for relaxation 39
    tissue 63

Water 25, 28, 32, 33, 78, 108, 147, 172, 255
    binding 256
    content 29
    levels 258
    retention 200
Waterman, Ian 42
Wave structure 63, 78, 80, 85
Weight 171, 192, 198
Whole-body
    coordination 86
    exercise(s) 107, 227
    movement 77, 92, 232
    training 106
    vibration 225
Woman 114, 116, 119, 132, 196, 199, 200,
    202, 247, 258, 267
Wound 48, 53, 84, 105, 115, 121
    healing 35, 43, 113, 118, 235, 247, 257,
    258, 260
Wrist 202

Y
Yoga 58, 77, 103, 231
    mat 119
    yin 235

Z
Zinc 257, 259